Sickle Cell Anemia: A Mother's Perspective

WHAT EVERY PARENT SHOULD KNOW

Sickle Cell Anemia: A Mother's Perspective

TABLE OF CONTENTS

Forward

My Personal Reflections

Sickle Cell was there but I did not know it. I had this uneasy feeling of "something" being present. Was my bouncing baby girl blind? I find it hard to believe that 48 hours have passed and she has not yet opened her eyes, dismissing the ultra bright beaming hospital lights. Something was afoot……..but what?

A call from the pediatrician three weeks later confirmed my gut feeling of something being present; my baby was born with Sickle Cell Anemia, a chronic illness. Was this a death sentence? Well at the time I thought so. Little did I know that this would be our introduction to an over extended relationship with doctors, hospitals and intravenous needles. How did it happen? Why did this happen? What does having the disease really mean and most importantly—where do I go from here? Because the disease is so unpredictable I am not sure what the future of having Sickle Cell Anemia means for my child's health but I know that this will result in a lifetime of education for me.

In the blink of an eye, my normal life had been turned upside-down. Confusion plagued me, depression dominated my every feeling, but there was absolutely no room for powerlessness in my life. I was no stranger to struggle and yes, I was down but not out. Anxiety coupled with fear, ignorance and pain initially crippled my thought processes but did not succeed in robbing me of my sanity. While dealing with the initial shock and various emotions, I knew that it was imperative that I learn about this pain crippling disease and quick. I knew that having self-pity and feeling sorry for my child would be nothing more than a detriment to her health and possibly the source of her demise. So what was a mother to do? Well, I can tell you what this mother did—I dug deep, brushed my shoulders off, and tapped into every possible source of knowledge—textbooks, articles, the National Institute of Health, blogs, available researchers,

Hematologists and other mothers of children with the disease. I left no stone unturned.

When your child is chronically ill, there is so much to learn. Because your child is newly diagnosed there will be lots of "trial and error." This is my reason for writing this book. I am hopeful that other parents of children living with Sickle Cell Disease will use this book as a learning tool and also to familiarize themselves with situations that they are bound to encounter. There are so many parents that take what a Professional tells them to be gospel without further researching. I am neither dismissing the credentials of the Professionals nor implying that what they are saying is false. My bottom line is that parents know their child better than anyone.

My Information & Sources

The information provided is based on my personal experiences coupled with direction from various physicians located in upstate New York. According to the US Census Bureau the total population of the County in which we reside is 298,130. The population is comprised of 81.8% Caucasian and 12.3% African American. Why is this relevant? I believe this information is relevant because the population is predominantly Caucasian and Sickle Cell Disease is overwhelmingly characterized as a disease which primarily affects the African American population. It is my personal opinion that Sickle Cell Disease is not very high on the medical community's priority list in this area.

We may as well address this issue right from the start. There will be times when you will encounter discrimination, indifference, possibly even racism. Those are ugly words but the reality is they exist in our world and you need to be prepared to combat them. Recently, the hospital in which my child receives care was allegedly providing disparate treatment when caring for patients of color. [1] In addition, I believe some of the Hematologists have limited backgrounds working primarily with pediatric Sickle Cell patients.

[1] http://www.timesunion.com/AspStories/story.asp?storyID=923166&category=STATE

The clinic where my child receives care primarily treats patients predominantly diagnosed with cancer and leukemia; sickle cell seems to be just there, out on the perimeter if you will. As a result, you may experience instances where you're left feeling your child has been slighted; your child may feel it too. For example, there's a particular organization that serves as one of the funding sources to provide book bags and school supplies to the children diagnosed with cancer and leukemia. Now I would be remiss if I did not add children with sickle cell do reap some benefits, which includes receiving toys during wellness visits or receiving gifts at Christmas time. Further, in the past if there was a surplus of school supplies my child did receive a book bag. There have also been times when I was told that the book bags were donated by a certain organization for specific diagnosis, so therefore, the book bags were for those children. So, despite the shortcomings and considering the availability of hospitals in our county, I am convinced that I have chosen the best hospital/clinic in my area to provide care for my child.

There is Nothing Like Getting the First-Hand Perspective

There are many books available that will explain the formal medical perspective on sickle cell anemia. There is also information available from Organizations that offer an accurate account of the disease; however, hearing about a mother's plight straight from the mother's mouth is totally different. As a mother, I have learned a lot of information from practitioners and by reading books. I also learned a lot about sickle cell disease through "trial and error." I would have personally appreciated a book like this when my child was first diagnosed.

I Refuse to be "Lost in Emotion"

As time has progressed I was at odds with myself about writing this book. I just didn't know if I wanted to share my child's medical issues with the entire world. Some people I spoke with wanted to know what the big deal was. The big deal is that my child has a right to privacy and if she wants to talk about her medical information, she can. Was it fair of me to just blurt everything out? To be honest, I still feel uneasy over doing this, however, I have gained such a wealth of information in the process of caring for my child that I may be able to prevent another mother from experiencing undue stress. I am not a weak person in any sense of the word, neither am I easily frightened or intimidated by events life throws at me. Now, I am not saying that I'm some kind of warrior, but I come pretty damn close! Actually, I am human and as such I am prone to bouts of confusion, depression, frustration, you name it! However, I cannot afford to wallow in those emotions because my child's health and well-being are at stake. Instead, I rise to the challenges that confront me and meet them head-on. Many mothers just now facing the devastating news that their child has sickle cell anemia may not be able to rise to the challenge---yet! I cannot erase the sense of devastation those mothers feel but with the information provided; I may be able to help them through their lifelong journey.

You Don't Know the Pain I Feel

Why me? We learn that we shouldn't answer a question with a question, but as time has progressed I found the answer to this question to be, Why not me? There is a prevailing message throughout the Sickle Cell community, which is *"you don't know the pain I feel."* This message rings true. A person that hasn't been diagnosed with Sickle Cell Anemia would not know or be able to imagine the physical pain experienced by this population. Yes, it's true, however, there is a pain that we parent's feel having a child diagnosed with Sickle Cell. The emotional pain is a pain that never leaves you, it is a constant companion. Just knowing that your child can experience physical pain at any time and there is nothing that can be done to stop it. Knowing that someday your child may need to take several narcotics just to maintain is a hurting feeling. Watching an intravenous needle being placed in your infant child's tiny arm and hearing your child yelling, "please, help me, "is a horrible feeling. Looking up at the IV pole only to notice that a stranger's blood is running through my child's veins makes your heart ache. The worst feeling in the world is to know that your child has a shortened life expectancy; however, there is hope in stem cell research and medications. What do you do? You make the most of it! While in your child's presence you have to keep your game face on because you want your child to know that you have their back and that everything is going to be ok. They see you cry, it makes them feel worse. My message to the Sickle Cell community is *"you don't know the pain we parents feel!"*

The Purpose of this Book

The purpose of this book is to chronicle the first seven years of our journey into the realm of sickle cell disease, what we have learned , how we have coped, and to provide information and guidance on what we have gleaned along the way.

The medical professionals in your lives are experts at what they do so please don't lose sight of that. I offer my personal advice on medical situations that I have experienced. Remember, it is just my advice and what worked for me. I am not a medical professional nor do I claim to be. Yes, I do have a few letters of the alphabet following my name but I assure you, no combination of those letters equal "MD." On the other hand, no combination of those letters spells out "dummy" either! As you read about some of my situations you will understand what I mean.

With having parental expertise and a medical professional at your side, your child can do great. I am also encouraging parents/caretakers to ask questions and not be afraid to. Don't bow down in the face of intimidation for it will only silence you. Finally, I want to emphasize that every parent/caretaker must learn everything possible about this disease. You are your child's superhero and advocate. They need you. Don't ever give up!

Diagnosis Sickle Hell!!!!

What is Sickle Cell Anemia or Hemoglobin SS (hbss) disease?

Sickle cell anemia is an inherited blood disorder distinguished by chronic anemia, sporadic pain events commonly known as "crisis," and various complications associated with tissue and organ damage. A person with Sickle Cell Anemia creates defective hemoglobin. After the hemoglobin molecules releases their oxygen into the tissues, some may cluster together causing the red blood cells to become stiff, hard, and sticky, forming in a sickle shape. Unlike normal red cells, which are smooth with a round shape, the sickled red cells cannot squeeze through small blood vessels. As a result of the sickled blood cells being restricted, they are unable to bring oxygen to the tissues of the body causing pain and damage to the affected areas leading to serious medical problems.[2] Sickle cells have a decreased life span in comparison to normal red blood cells. Normal red blood cells survive for approximately 120 days in the bloodstream and sickled cells last only 10-20 days. Consequently, the blood stream is chronically short of red blood cells and hemoglobin resulting in the individual developing anemia.[3]

How is Sickle Cell Diagnosed?

Typically sickle cell anemia is diagnosed at birth with a simple blood test. This is done in combination with other routine newborn screening tests. Hemoglobin electrophoresis is the most commonly used diagnostic test. If your child tests positive on the screening test, a second blood test usually is completed to confirm the diagnosis. Due to the increased risk of infection in children with sickle cell anemia early diagnosis and treatment is imperative. Presently, more than 40 states have newborn screening programs for sickle cell anemia.

---

[2] National Institute of Health. NIH Publication No. 96-4057. November 1996.

[3] http://www.myoptumhealth.com/portal/DiseasesandConditions/item/Sickle+cell+disease

What causes Sickle Cell Anemia?

Sickle Cell Anemia is a genetic blood disorder passed from parent to child. It is caused by an error in the gene that tells the body how to make hemoglobin. The faulty gene instructs the body to make the defective hemoglobin that results in abnormal red blood cells. A child must inherit two defective hemoglobin S genes, one from each parent, to be born with Sickle Cell Anemia. The gene for sickle cell anemia is more common in African Americans and people from the Mediterranean countries, the Middle East, and India. According to the Center for Disease Control and Prevention and the National Heart Lung and Blood Institute Disease and Conditions Index, "In the United States, it's estimated that sickle cell anemia affects 70k-100k people, mainly African Americans. The disease occurs in about 1 out of every 500 African American births. Sickle cell anemia also affects Hispanic Americans. The disease occurs in 1 out of every 36k Hispanic American births. About 2 million Americans have sickle cell trait. The condition occurs in about 1 in 12 African Americans."

Sickle What????? I Don't Understand the Technical Talk- I Need a Layman's Explanation ....

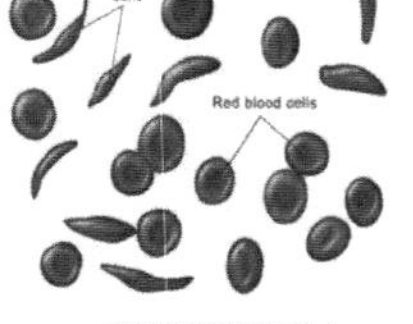

I knew of Sickle Cell. I always associated it with lots of pain without ever thinking about the cause. Well that has changed! I now needed to know what exactly was going on inside my child's body. My child would be subjected to pain, but why? I had not taken Biology or Chemistry since high school (I will just say some time ago LOL). I began searching the Internet for information and found lots of it. I never made the mistake of believing everything that I read on the Internet. I am one of those people who digs, digs and digs. The information that I found to be trustworthy came from reliable sources such as the National Institute of Health. Further research took me to the Sickle Cell Disease Association of America, Inc. With my ongoing research I found out what was going on inside my child's body. I found several explanations. The easiest way for me to understand what was going on inside was to imagine that I was trying to squeeze the moon through a straw. Obviously the moon is not a perfect fit, however, I can shove the moon inside the straw because the edges are smooth and circular. Think of this as being the normal red blood cell flowing through the blood vessel. Now let's pretend that we are trying to do the same thing with a crescent instead of the moon. . Both ends of the crescent are not smooth and very pointy. How much success would we have getting a crescent through the straw? Not much! Again, we try stuffing the crescent through the straw but have no success because both ends are sharp and sticky. We force and force, however, we continue to have a hard time. Because the ends are sharp and sticky there is resistance when trying to force it through. This symbolizes the oxygen deprived sticky sickled cell that is stuck at some area in the body (can be anywhere) and will not move smoothly. The crescent is stuck and there are a million other crescents coming behind it. Where the crescent is stuck symbolizes how sickled cells cause pain [4]crisis. This can be the beginning of a pain crisis. The sickled cell starts out round and due to defective hemoglobin it changes into a sickled shape. A picture of this sickling process can be found at the Medical College of Georgia's website.[5]

I hope that my layman's explanation helped you to grasp some understanding of how sickled cells can cause pain.

The National Institute of Health's Professional Explanation of Sickle Cell Disease

As one can imagine, there is an official medical explanation that describes what sickle cell is and how this disease functions inside the body. The best factually based explanation I've discovered comes from the National Institute of Health. Just keep my layman's explanation in mind and it should not be complicated to understand the official technical medical explanation.

"Sickle Cell anemia (uh-NEE-me-uh) is a serious disease in which the body makes sickle-shaped red blood cells. "Sickle-shaped" means that the red blood cells are shaped like a "C."Normal red blood cells are disc-shaped and look like doughnuts without holes in the center. They move easily through your blood vessels. Red blood cells contain the protein hemoglobin (HEE-muh-glow-bin). This iron-rich protein gives blood its red color and carries oxygen from the lungs to the rest of the body. Sickle Cells contain abnormal hemoglobin that causes the cells to have a sickle shape. Sickle-shaped cells don't move easily through your blood vessels. They're stiff and sticky and tend to form clumps and get stuck in the blood vessels. (Other cells also may play a role in this clumping process.)The clumps of Sickle Cells block blood flow in the blood

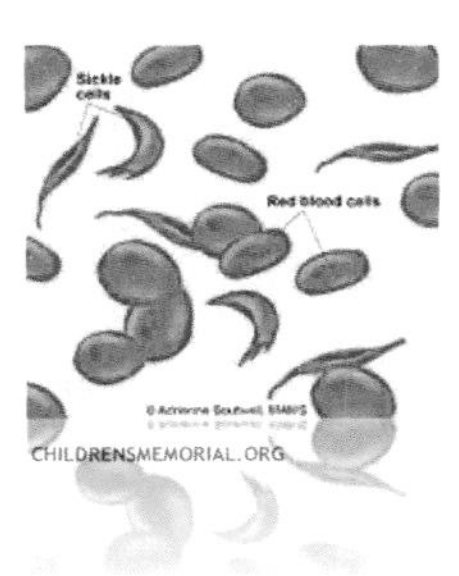

---

http://www.mcg.edu/centers/sicklecell/

vessels that lead to the limbs and organs. Blocked blood vessels can cause pain, serious infections, and organ damage."

Your Next Move: Keep Moving Forward!

Educating Yourself Immediately

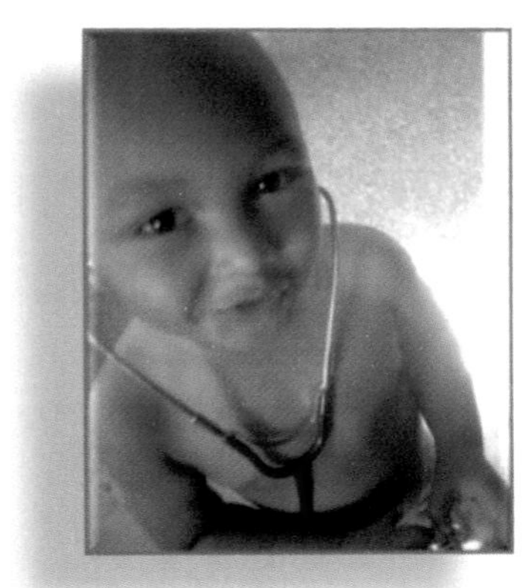

As soon as you receive the call from your Pediatrician's office informing you that your child's New Born Screening test should be repeated because it looks like your child may have Sickle Cell Disease, you must begin to prepare for the diagnosis.

I know this is easier said than done. Subsequent to your being informed that your child may soon be diagnosed with a painful chronic illness, it may be a bit difficult to function. The feeling of instability comes quick followed by utter confusion without having a clue as to what to do. This is why I am writing this, to offer suggestions and direction at a time when you may make irrational emotional decisions.

Your child will be around 30 days old when you receive the first call from the Pediatrician and schedule for the confirmation testing to be completed. You can ask your Pediatrician to refer you to a Pediatric Hematologist who has experience managing Sickle Cell Disease. When this information is provided, schedule an appointment with the Pediatric Hematology Oncology Office for a consult and initial visit. They will ask if you're a new patient and want to know what 's going on. Inform the receptionist of the phone call you received from the

Pediatrician and explain that you would like to have confirmation testing completed. They are going to get you in quick.

The diagnosis hasn't been formally confirmed until a second round of testing has been completed. Once your child receives a formal diagnosis, you will not be able to purchase a life insurance policy because companies will deny the child due to preexisting condition. As of present, you just received the call informing you that your child "may" have Sickle Cell Disease and additional testing is required to confirm, therefore, your child has not been formally diagnosed. If you have not purchased a life insurance policy for your child, this may not be a bad time to look into purchasing one.

The First Pediatric Hematology Appointment

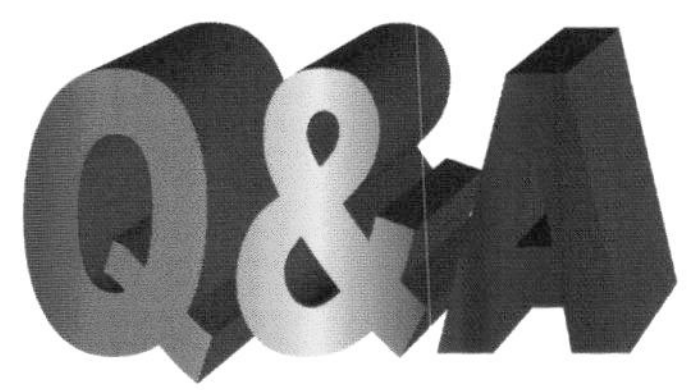

You are probably nervous and unsure of what to expect. There are a few things that you can do to prepare. If possible both parents and/or caregivers should attend this appointment. This is going to be important because this appointment is going to be more "informational" than anything. This is going to be the appointment to cry at and have the Q&A session. This is not the time to point fingers and place blame on anyone for the child having this disease. This is the time to move forward and learn about the child's disease, how best to take care of him/her and to learn strategies that will ensure comfort for your child at all times. You will receive tons of information so don't forget to bring a pen and notebook to this appointment. You can also write some questions that you may have before arriving.

Questions you want to ask include, but are not limited to:

- ✓ How long has the doctor been working with Sickle Cell patients?
- ✓ What to expect with this disease?
- ✓ How often will the Hematologist have to see you?
- ✓ What is a pain crisis?
- ✓ At what age should you expect to see a pain crisis?
- ✓ What is the doctor's policy on fevers? How high should the fever be before your child will have to be admitted or seen in the ER?
- ✓ You want to ask what type of Sickle Cell your child has, although that will not be determined until your child completes further blood testing
- ✓ You want to know the recommended fluid intake for your child
- ✓ Ask for information that you can take home and read

- ✓ You want to know the on call procedures
- ✓ Ask how many Hematologists work in the clinic and how many will be working with your child and what are their specialties (your Hematologist will not be working every day all year, so there will be others)

At this appointment and every future appointment, your child will be getting blood drawn. The electrophoresis test will be completed and will provide the confirmation that your child does indeed have Sickle Cell Disease and the type. Although the child is being tested a second time to confirm the diagnosis, the child will still be treated as a child already diagnosed.

What to Expect at Your Routine Hematology Appointments(s)

Complete Blood Count (CBC)

Your child will need to be seen by his/her hematologist every 3 months. At each visit expect that your child will have a Complete Blood Count (CBC) completed. This test gives the doctor information on your child's current status. What I learned from the practice of my child's Hematologist (30+ years experience) is that the CBC does not have to be collected via vein. It can be collected with a simple finger stick. The doctor's rationale was that if the child's vein did not have to be used he wasn't going to use it. He explained to me that this is a lifelong disease and my child would need her veins to be maintained in the best condition (as possible) for as long as possible. I understood and actually appreciated his reasoning. But what you have to beware of is that this may not be routine practice by every Hematologist or phlebotomist. The RN's will tell you that they never heard of taking blood for a CBC through a finger stick or they don't do it that way. They will tell you that the blood is going to coagulate and will not be good for testing. Don't believe the hype, it can be done. What they should say is that they graduated from school so long ago and don't have the experience to keep it from clotting. What I learned as a parent is that many of these phlebotomists and

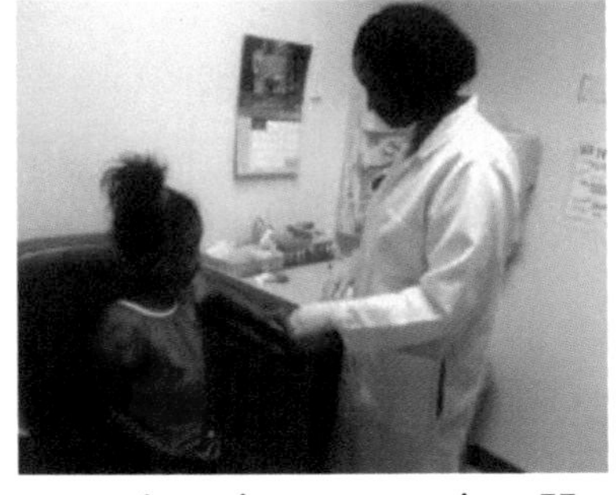

nurses find it easier to use the vein. It takes a very special phlebotomist to collect a finger stick correctly and keep it from clotting. Depending on the season, be sure that your child's hands are warm. They will be able to collect the amount they need and then some. Remember, you are your child's best advocate, you are a part of the child's medical team and you have the final say. I happen to be the mother that doesn't intimidate easily and I will not just go with the flow of things because it is comfortable for others. Your child's well-being and comfort come first. FYI: there will be times when the Hematologist will need a good amount of blood and a finger stick will not suffice. These are the times when the veins should be used. Just my opinion!

Medications Prescribed for your Child

Your Hematologist will prescribe and review medications during routine appointments. At your initial appointment your child may be prescribed two medications. The medications will be prescribed according to age and risk. The medications that will be prescribed are Penicillin VK and 1mg of Folic Acid.

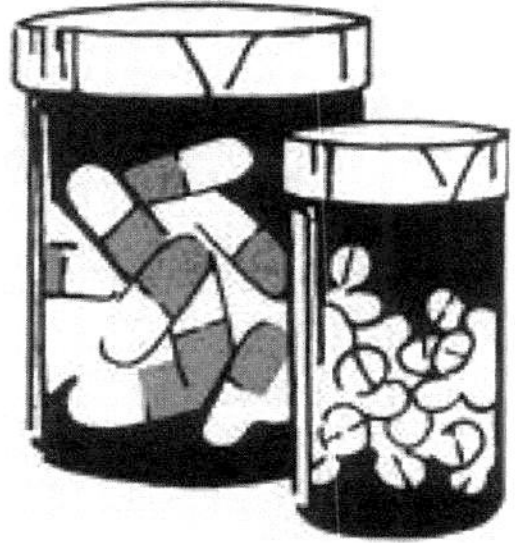

MEDBOTTLE.CT.GOV

You're probably wondering why your child would need to be prescribed prophylactic penicillin and the duration in which your child is expected to take it. According to the National Institute of Health, "**penicillin** markedly reduces the incidence of pneumococcal sepsis." I also found a second site that spells it out in a way that everyone can easily understand. The quick penicillin facts are below:

- ✓ Infection in the bloodstream is the leading cause of death in young children with Sickle Cell disease
- ✓ Taking penicillin by mouth 2 times a day every day can greatly decrease the risk of infection in the bloodstream
- ✓ Your child's best defense to prevent bloodstream infections is to take penicillin 2 times a day every day
- ✓ Penicillin should be started by 2 - 3 months of age, and stopped by your child's physician, usually by age 5 years
- ✓ Liquid penicillin is often easier to give young children, but is also available in tablet form

- ✓ Liquid penicillin must be stored in the refrigerator and it must not be kept for longer than 2 weeks
- ✓ Liquid penicillin should be measured using a dosing syringe, given to you by your nurse or pharmacist. Do not use a kitchen teaspoon because it is not accurate
- ✓ Penicillin tablets should be stored in a cool, dry place. Tablets may be kept as long as 4 months
- ✓ Don't take a chance with your child's health; give penicillin 2 times a day, every day

The Penicillin will be prescribed as a prophylactic from the time of diagnosis (roughly 2-3months old). From diagnosis to age 3 your child will have to take 125mg twice daily. At age 3 to 5 your child's dose will be increased to 250mg twice daily. In some instances you are given the option to keep your child on the Penicillin until age 6. I was given this option and decided against it. I feared that my child would become resistant to antibiotic treatment.

The second medication that your child will be prescribed is 1mg of folic acid. Your child will need to take 1 pill daily for the rest of his/her life. The folic acid is a vitamin B supplement that is necessary in aiding the body in the consistent creation of new red blood cells. The red blood cells in Sickle patients are destroyed and/or break down quickly (10-20 days) in comparison to an individual living without the disease (120 days) as previously discussed on page 1. As always, educate yourself about the known side effects of each medication.

The Physical Exam

The Hematologist will then conduct a physical exam. The child will have his/her height, weight, and oxygen levels taken. The doctor will ask if the child has had any fevers, fatigue or pain. Your Hematologist will also review the immunizations ensuring that they are up to date. S/he will also inquire to see if you have any questions, comments or concerns.

Immunizations

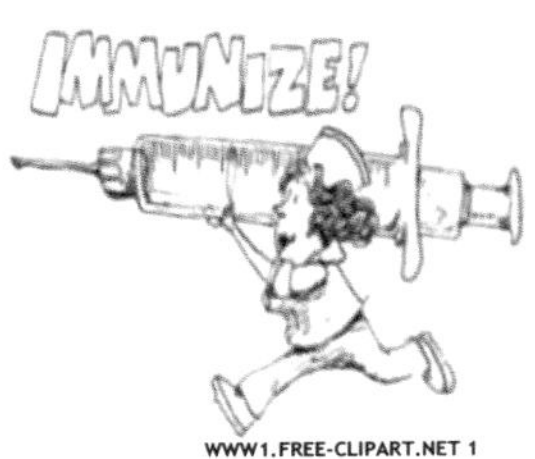

Vaccines serve to prevent and protect everyone from malicious diseases. There is a recommended vaccination schedule for every child, however, children diagnosed with Sickle Cell Disease need a few extra in addition to the regularly scheduled vaccines. According to the Center for Disease Control the extra vaccines are:

- ✓ *Flu vaccine (influenza vaccine) every year after 6 months of age.*
- ✓ *A special pneumococcal vaccine (called 23-valent pneumococcal vaccine) at 2 and 5 years of age.*
- ✓ *Meningococcal vaccine, if recommended by a doctor.* [3]

If your child is not up-to-date, they will give the shots right then and there.

Visit & Educational Review

Before the conclusion of the visit the Hematologist will provide general information such as strategies that you can use to keep your child well at home. S/he will discuss hydration, pain management, fever and environment. The Hematologist will also discuss specific information about your child such as a review of the current CBC count and what the counts indicate. S/he will also discuss what symptoms to look for at this particular time. S/he should also give you specific instructions on how to contact the office after hours should your child become sick or other concerns you may have. This will conclude your visit. When checking out, be sure to schedule your next appointment.

The "In's and Out's" of the Routine Visit....My 2 Cents

Now that I pretty much shared an overview of what happens during a routine hematology visit, I am going to share little tips that I learned over the years.

- ✓ Always document what occurs on a routine hematology visit. You want to write down what happened (what the hematologist did, any medications prescribed with dose), when it happened (date of visit), where did the visit occur (clinic or emergency room), who attended the visit (you, name of hematologist, nurse), and why were you at this visit. Believe me, your record keeping will come in handy over the years.
- ✓ At every visit they will discuss the results of the CBC. Always obtain a copy of the report for yourself. You want to be on the same page as the Hematologist.

- ✓ Be sure to always ask questions if you are not sure about something. Do not be afraid or embarrassed. It is imperative that you learn about what is going on with your child. It is vital that you are able to recognize the first signs of a crisis.
- ✓ Sometimes the hematologist will decide a certain course of care regarding your child. Do not stand there like a ham sandwich and just agree without understanding why the hematologist chose that particular course of care. . Find out why they are choosing the course of care. Ask questions and keep asking questions until you fully understand. Sometimes the Hematologist will get frustrated and feel that you are questioning their intelligence. You are merely learning from their intelligence.
- ✓ Before you leave the office know all about the on-call, you may have to use it. Know the number to the clinic by heart. You're probably thinking if my child gets sick I am going to the ER. I understand that it is a parent's instinct to be sure that their child is ok. There is benefit to using the hematology on-call after hours. For one, if the child has a high fever or is in extreme pain, the hematologist is able to obtain a hospital room faster than you would by going through the Emergency Room. Further, the hematologist is familiar with your child and has a better idea of what is going on. Make no mistake about it, there will be times that you must use the ER and your parental instincts coupled with your ongoing education about the disease will let you know when that is.
- ✓ Ask what type of Sickle Cell your child has. Be sure to ask what the difference is between your child's Sickle Cell type and other types. This information is very important. You will need to know the type when learning about signs, symptoms, fevers and pain management.
- ✓ Ask the hematologist for information explaining your child's disease. It is now your duty to learn and read everything –even those things you "think" are unimportant.

Hematologist, Phlebotomist & Other Scary Names

Up until now most of your experiences with those in the medical profession likely centered around a family doctor, pediatrician, gynecologist, and dentist. Then you have a child diagnosed with sickle cell disease. Suddenly you find yourself listening to your pediatrician and you're being told to set up an appointment with Hematology/Oncology clinic and the very sound of those words strikes fear in your heart. I assure you, there is nothing to fear from those scary sounding names. These are Specialists trained in specific fields who will be providing specialized treatment and care for your child. You should familiarize yourself with them and their specialties.

Not So Scary Names

Hematologist- expert in blood disorders

Phlebotomist- expert at drawing blood

Pulmonologist- expert at treating diseases of the lungs

Cardiologist-expert of the heart

Stat Nurse-expert at drawing blood, this nurse is usually called when every other attempt has failed in someway

Pediatrician, Hematologist & Other Members of your child's Medical Team—Distinguish the Roles!!!!!!

A child diagnosed with Sickle Cell disease will have several doctors in his/her life . As your child ages and begins to have various complications there will be more doctors joining the team. So let's take a closer look at the doctors. It is very important that you are able to distinguish the roles of all doctors that will be involved in your child's life. This was very confusing for me, however I began to differentiate roles and duties fast. . The confusion began for me with the role of the primary care physician and the Hematologist. Read on, you will soon understand why.

Your child will have a primary care physician (PCP) also known as a family doctor to provide basic care such as immunizations, treat ear infections, conduct annual physical exams and for the most part, preventative care. Your primary doctor is trained to treat a variety of health issues and is responsible for the child's continuous care. Your PCP, primary doctor and Pediatrician are one in the same. Pediatricians specialize in the health care of infants through young adult. Think of your PCP as your second line of defense. You are the parent and your child's first line of defense! If your child has any type of issues going on including mental and/or physical, you are going to call to schedule an appointment with the PCP first. Now you must realize that there are going to be some medical issues that your Pediatrician can not treat; however, the Pediatrician is able to assess what is going on. If you have an issue that is beyond the scope of the Pediatrician's practice the Pediatrician will refer you to the appropriate Specialist. In the case of Sickle Cell Disease the appropriate Specialist is a Hematologist.

As I was told real simple, the Hematologist is the doctor that studies blood. For the purpose of this book the focus is on the Hematologist and his/her role with my child, a pediatric Sickle Cell patient. The Hematologist is a huge part of your child's medical team. I will take it a step further and say that the Hematologist is the primary part and most important part of your child's team. Yes, I know I just had that big monologue going on about the role of the PCP in the last paragraph. But remember, I also said that the roles can become confusing. Welcome to the land of confusion! LOLLLL

What I found confusing at first is that my child's Hematologist functioned as her primary doctor as well as the role intended. I didn't question it because it was more convenient than not.

Most of the time, I found that my child's Hematologist was pretty much doing everything including immunizations, physicals, and prescribing medicine. I am thinking, cool! One particular year I needed the Hematologist to complete the annual physical for school. This particular year the Hematologist told me to schedule an appointment with my PCP. I asked her why since she had been pretty much functioning as the PCP. She told me that annual physicals should be completed with the PCP. Well what could I do? I had not been to see the PCP in so long I had to find my Provider Directory for the insurance company. Along with the directory I found the Members Handbook. I had never read it and the best place I thought for it was the trash. As I walked to the trashcan I began to wonder what is actually in it. So I took what I thought was going to be a quick peek. I skim through the first few pages when suddenly I came across valuable information. Well low and behold, look what I have here! Wanna take a guess? I found a section that read as follows, , *" You may be able to choose a specialist to act as your PCP. You might be able to do this if you have a long-lasting illness like HIV?AIDS or other long-term health problems."* I was so happy when I saw this. My Hematologist had been acting as the PCP anyway until now. I placed a call to my insurance company and had them switch my child's primary care to her Hematologist. I can tell you from personal experience, there are pros and no cons in doing this. The pros are that your Hematologist becomes your one-stop-shop. Everything is done through your Hematologist. This combined role will eliminate waiting periods for your Hematologist and PCP to communicate, the confusion that will arise with immunizations and your Hematologist will be the first to know about all emergencies that may arise.

Other Specialist's "may" join your child's medical team. You notice I said, "may" right? This doesn't mean they will have to. You may likely have other medical professionals that work with your child as well. Children with Sickle Cell are treated according to the health issues that arise. So it is important to become familiar with the different type of Specialists and their functions.

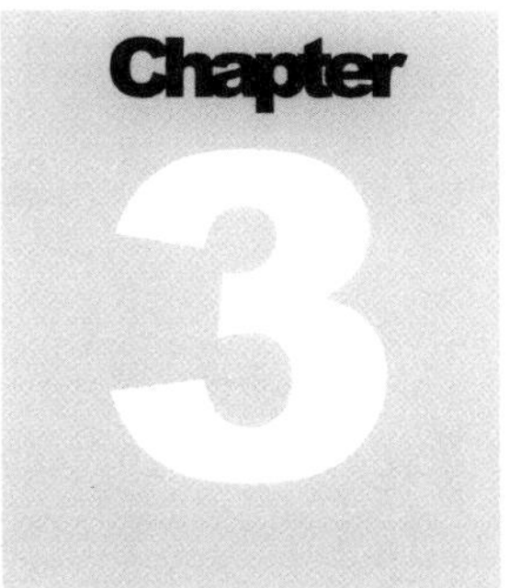

Parenting & Managing Sickle Cell Disease at Home

Managing Sickle Cell Disease at Home One day at a Time!

What you need to know

- ✓ How to recognize when your child is getting sick
- ✓ The sickle cell preventative tools
- ✓ Have Hematologist's phone number on speed dial

What you need to do

- ✓ *Use your Sickle Cell Crisis Prevention Strategies*

  As discussed, your Hematologist will provide information that will assist you in caring for your child at home and which could possibly impede or prevent a crisis. Learn the basics of prevention techniques and in the long run you will develop your own strategies to strengthen and complement the prevention tools given by the Hematologist.

- ✓ *Always Comfort your Child*

  Be sure that your child is receiving enough fluids, is dressed appropriately, eating healthy food, taking medicines as prescribed, gets plenty of rest, and not engaging in strenuous activities. These tasks are easier said than done; however, you can do it. The constant battle in my home has been getting my child to drink enough fluids.

First Crisis: Paranoid Panicked Parent Mode

There is a level of comfort while in the presence of a hematologist. You have that comfort because if something goes wrong the hematologist will handle it. When you have to take your child home and something goes wrong for the first time, it is very scary. This is when the paranoid panicked parent mode kicked into high gear for me. Not knowing what to expect or when to expect it is horrible!. Expecting the worst was easy and made me nervous all the time. I began to hate the element of surprise. I had already read the "what could" happen list but wasn't as focused on prevention. My best advice for the paranoid panic parent is to focus on the "prevention" of an episode. Will you always be able to prevent every episode? No you will not! This does not mean that you become relaxed when putting the preventative tools to use. These are the very tools that your hematologist should have given you by now. These are the things that you can do at home to bring comfort to your child. One thing you must recognize is that your child knows when you are worried, nervous or sad. You're the protector; their confidence in you must not be shaken. In short, when you are around your child you must keep your game face on even when you're feeling hollow inside. This will let your child know that you are there for them and everything is going to be alright.

Learned Tips for managing Sickle Cell at home:

Preventative Tools Defined

Hydration → You must keep your child hydrated. Be sure that s/he drinks plenty of fluids throughout the course of the day. Sickled Cells are sticky and drinking lots of fluid help the sticky cells move throughout the body. As your child gets older hydration will certainly become a struggle and you as a parent must stand your ground and be firm. Remember a lack of fluids will almost guarantee a hospital stay. How much should you child drink? The rule of thumb is, when your child urinates, s/he must take a drink to replace the voided fluid.

Rest→ It is expected that your child will be more fatigued than the average child his/her age. Be sure that your child is well rested and is allowed as many breaks throughout the day as needed when s/he feels tired.

Oxygen→ Be sure that your child is breathing clean air. Your child should not be in an atmosphere where people are smoking. If there is a smoker in the house, s/he should be made to smoke outside of the house or quit. This may sound farfetched to a smoker but it shouldn't- your child's life depends on it. Also be careful that your child does not participate in overly strenuous activities that could cause a loss of oxygen, (like running).

Hand Washing→ Practice hand-washing, lots of hand washing. There are so many germs your child is being exposed to and germs seem to be getting stronger than ever. I was told by a nurse that some exposure to germs are good because your child may possibly build a resistance, however, for every good exposure there are ten nasty germs. Your child must wash their hands regularly.

Heating Pad→ A heating pad may ease the pain. Always have one available at home. Always follow the manufacturer's directions that accompany the heating pad.

Prescribed Medications→ Be sure that your child is taking all prescribed medications as directed. I cannot stress how important it is that you develop and maintain a consistent medication regimen. There is a reason why your child is prescribed these medications. Yes, the medication is going to be long term and you may even be tired of running to the drug store and remembering when to give your child his/her meds. I say, "so what if you're tired!" Your child needs his/her meds to stay well, be sure that s/he gets them.

Do Not Forget→ There is a chance that your child may experience pain while at home. Be sure that you get a prescription for Tylenol 3 (also known as Codeine) to keep at home. This will help you to keep a pain crisis under control and/or buy time so that you will be able to get to the hospital. You must request this medication from your Hematologist, however, s/he may offer it.

Avoid, Avoid, Avoid!

As your Hematologist should have told you, there are several situations that you want to steer clear of. These situations include but are not limited to:

Extreme hot and cold temperatures→ The biggest mistake that parents tend to make is to overdress their children. You should dress your child as you dress yourself. If you are going outside and only wearing a sweater your child should not be wearing a coat.

Avoid swimming in unheated pools. I learned that unheated water tends to be too cold and "cold" causes pain crisis in children with Sickle Cell.

Avoid travel on unpressurized airplanes At first it wasn't clear as to why my child should not fly in an unpressurized plane so I began to ask questions and search around. Planes fly at altitudes where oxygen levels are diminished and the higher the altitude the lower the oxygen level becomes. As you've learned by now, Sickle Cell is a disease characterized by oxygen deprivation resulting in pain. If you must travel a long distance on a plane in altitudes above 8000 feet and your child is traveling with you, be sure to consult with your child's Hematologist first. Flying at high altitude for anyone diagnosed with Sickle Cell disease is very dangerous and has serious health consequences. Consulting with your child's Hematologist before flying is not optional, it's a must! Your child's life depends on it!

Be On the Lookout For…

The Freauent Fevers & Infection

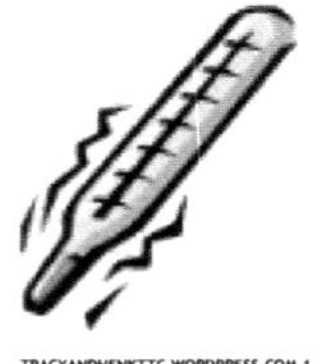

TRACYANDHENKTTC.WORDPRESS.COM 1

What you need to Know

- ✓ How to recognize that your child has a fever (symptoms)
- ✓ You need to know your child's baseline temperature
- ✓ Your Hematologist's protocol to follow when your child becomes febrile (hot, inflamed, fevered)
- ✓ At what temperature does your Hematologist consider the child's fever dangerous

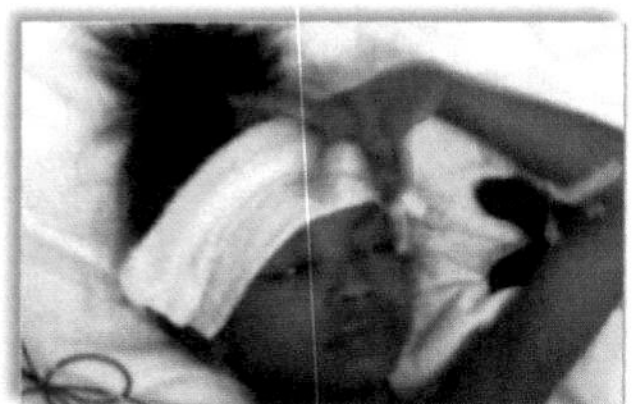

What you need to do

Comfort your child (do not wrap your child in blankets)

Be sure that your child is not over dressed. Have your child sit or lay down in a comfortable place. Offer and continue to reinforce fluids. Your child may not feel like drinking anything or may even refuse. Refusal is not an option. Your child must continue to sip or drink fluids.

Review the child's symptoms and determine if the symptoms are consistent with fever?

Fever is a sign that "something is going on inside the body" and in the case of children diagnosed with Sickle Cell, fever is a sign of infection (bacterial or viral). Signs of fever may include; but are not limited to your child having a temperature greater than 101.0, has the chills, suddenly becomes very tired, chapped lips, cranky or any other uncharacteristic behavior. You know your child and you know when something is not right. Believe it or not intuition will kick in, don't ignore it!

Contact your child's Hematologist immediately. If it is after office hours, contact the on-call services and ask that the on call Hematologist call you immediately.

When the Hematologist returns your call you want to tell them everything that is going on. Express your concerns and ask them how they want you to proceed. Most likely they are going to instruct you to bring the child in. If it is during clinical hours they may have you bring the child in immediately and treat the child in the clinic with an antibiotic by IV and send you back home. If it is after hours they may have you bring the child straight to the Pediatric unit to be admitted (depending on current bed availability) or if there is no bed available, they will have you bring the child to the Emergency Room so treatment can begin and will admit the child as soon as a bed opens.

Be sure to document this fever in your medical journal and if you must take a trip to the hospital (likely) be sure that you have your medical journal with you.

As always, document everything that goes on with your child related to his/her illness. This is a good reference for you and certainly a good tool that will assist in your answering questions regarding your child's past treatment.

My Personal Issue

When my child becomes ill she needs treatment without question. What I find unsettling is that if my child falls ill during clinical hours I am instructed to bring her in to the clinic , they treat her and send her home. They give her Tylenol and Ibuprofen for fever with an IV antibiotic for the underlying infection that may be the source of the fever. After treatment we are sent home and guess what happens in a few hours? My child's fever spikes again and usually it's higher than the initial spike. So here we go again, I have to contact on-call service and receive instructions to bring my child back in. I don't care about having to go back but I do care about my child being stuck with needles 100 times (exaggeration) when they could have just admitted her the first time. Now she has to get yet another IV before finally being admitted. I understand that getting tons of needles is part of the treatment for Sickle Cell but aren't there ways to lessen this? I share this because it is my belief; if my child happens to have an emergency during clinical hours and has to receive an IV, I request that she be admitted. I damn near insist that they admit her. I feel the full course of treatment should be provided then and not broken up into this "day-by-day" thing. Do I suggest you do what I do? That is a decision that you the parent has to make; however, my goal is not to steer anyone wrong!

Know all about Your Child's Low Grade Fevers, Fevers & Baseline Temperature

The hematologist told me that it would be a good idea to take my child's temperature every day, even when she is feeling well. Of course I am thinking, "what?" So he went on to say that taking my child's temperature daily will give me an idea of what her baseline (normal temperature) is. Knowing the baseline is important and helpful because it informs me of my child's normal temperature and any small increase beyond the norm would indicate that my child is getting sick. If she did not have the Sickle diagnosis the fever would not be that big of a deal, however, fever is the first sign that your child is falling ill. For instance, my child's baseline is 98.7. When I see a small increase to about

99.9 that would be considered a low-grade fever for her. The "low grade" fever basically represents that there is something going on, it's underlying and waiting to rear its ugly head. Sometimes the low-grade fever can be tricky and fluctuate. It is very important to monitor your child's temperature consistently once you notice that s/he has had a low-grade fever. It takes only minutes for your child's low-grade fever to elevate into a major fever (101.0+). I guess I will say that my knowing the baseline and recognizing low-grade fevers takes the "guess work" out of it (for me anyway). The moral of the story is that it is important to know your child's baseline temperature and to have a plan in place when your child has a low-grade fever. As a parent I want to stress that all children with Sickle Cell are not the same; however, they are very similar. It is vital that you never ever dismiss a low-grade fever as being nothing because it is something, and you must keep an eye on it and be ready to react when your child's fever spikes full swing!

What does a fever actually mean for my child?

Fevers can mean a few things to parents of children diagnosed with Sickle Cell disease. Fever usually means that the child has contracted a bacterial infection which can lead to a serious crisis if left untreated plus, a guaranteed hospital stay. Infectious bacteria will make your child very ill. Previously I mentioned prophylactic penicillin. The penicillin will help keep the bad bacteria under control, however, sometimes penicillin alone is not enough and your child will still develop a fever. When this happens you must contact your child's Hematologist immediately and get to the hospital. There have been times that I have made the call to the Hematologist while on my way to the hospital. . Again, no one knows your child better than you do. If you feel your child is too sick, the fever is quickly escalating or your child is in pain—LEAVE! This is where your cell phone will come in handy. Your Hematologist can call you back while you are on your way to the hospital.

Dehydration (Monitor at all Times)

What you need to know

The symptoms

What you need to do

Be able to recognize the symptoms

What is dehydration?

Dehydration occurs when the amount of fluid leaving the body is greater than what is being taken in.

How is dehydration treated?

With IV fluids and drinking fluids by mouth

Signs of Dehydration

- ✓ Decreased urine output
- ✓ Dry sticky mouth and sunken eyes
- ✓ Drowsiness
- ✓ Unable to cry tears
- ✓ Elevated Hemoglobin levels
- ✓ Dark urine is a huge sign

On a Personal Note….

Keeping my child hydrated has been one of the biggest battles in my home. It is very easy when they are an infant because they suck baby bottles. Once the child begins to age, it may become one of your biggest struggles. Children are not always thirsty and will sometimes refuse to drink when they are not. When they are very young (toddler-age 7), they may not understand why they should have to drink when they are not thirsty and further, no one else is doing it. You may have to develop some tricks to get the child to drink more. Please be aware, the more they drink, the more they will urinate, even at night time. It may possibly lead to bed wetting. If this occurs, you can ask the primary care provider or the hematologist to write a prescription for pull-ups or store brand equivalent. If the child is over age 3, the State insurance (Medicaid) will cover the cost of pull-ups. The store brands can be crappy, so when you request the script from the doctor, be sure that they write the name brand (Pull-ups) and at the bottom of the script they should fill in the "DAW" box. DAW means "dispense as written." If the doctor does not write DAW in the box on the bottom of the script, the pharmacy will fill the script with a generic brand.

Splenic Sequestration (Very Serious Crisis)

What you need to know

- ✓ How to recognize this dangerous and **potentially deadly crisis**!!!!!!!!!

What you need to do

- ✓ ***Learn about the spleen, it's function, and about the crisis itself***
  This crisis is dangerous, very dangerous! My best advice would be to learn about regular

spleen function first. Once you have some understanding of what regular spleen function is, it would be beneficial to learn everything you can about spleenic sequestration.

What is a spleen and how does it function?

The spleen is a soft, spongy organ about the size of a fist. It's located just under the rib cage on the left side. The spleens function is twofold. It scans blood that passes through it for infection. Some of the blood cells in the spleen will attack the origin of the infections. Also, the spleen filters blood to remove unwanted material such as defective cells.

What is a splenic sequestration or spleen crisis?

With sickle cell anemia the sickled cells sometimes become trapped in blood vessels inside the spleen and leading out of the spleen, which prevents the normal flow of the blood. Blood in turn becomes trapped inside the spleen instead of flowing through it. This is called sequestration resulting in a decline in the hemoglobin blood count coupled with an enlarging of the spleen. If the spleen rapidly enlarges along with a significant drop in the blood count, this is a serious and potentially life-threatening problem, which should be checked by a physician immediately. If the blood count is severely low due to sequestration, the individual will most likely be treated with blood transfusion therapy.

Recurrent episodes are common, and a splenectomy (removal of the spleen) is sometimes required. After the spleen is removed, the body loses some ability to fight infection. But within a short time, other organs usually compensate for the loss of the spleen. People without a spleen will need additional vaccinations to defend against three key types of bacteria:

- ✓ Haemophilus influenza type B
- ✓ Pneumococcus
- ✓ Meningococcus [6]

Splenic sequestration most commonly occurs in children between the ages of 6 months to 2 years old. After age five years, the spleen becomes smaller and in most cases it cannot enlarge any more. Children with Sickle C Disease usually experience this complication after the age of five years.[7]

Symptoms of "Splenic Sequestration

- ✓ Weakness

---

[6] http://www.mayoclinic.com/invoke.cfm?id=AN00615

[7] http://www.scinfo.org/childSSispleen.htm

- ✓ Irritability
- ✓ Unusual sleepiness
- ✓ Paleness
- ✓ Enlarged spleen
- ✓ Fast heart beat
- ✓ Pain in the left side of the abdomen

Any enlargement of the spleen must be monitored. Your Hematologist will teach you how to feel for the child's spleen during routine well -visits. It is important to know how the child's spleen usually feels so that when he/she appears to be getting sick, you will be able to feel the difference and/or measure the spleen to see if it is bigger.

How is Spleenic Sequestration treated?

Blood transfusions or splenctomy

Aplastic Crisis

What you need to know

- ✓ Recognize symptoms (itemized list follows)

What you need to do

- ✓ Call the Hematologist and get your child to the hospital

What is an Aplastic Crisis

An aplastic crisis is an infection in the bone marrow caused by parvovirus B19. It causes production of red blood cells to be shut down for 7-10 days. This means that red blood cells are not being made during this time. Since the red blood cells in children with sickle cell anemia live only 10-15 days compared to 120 days in children who do not have sickle cell anemia, the hemoglobin count falls rapidly to dangerously low levels during the infection. A shortage of red blood cells may cause fatigue, paleness in appearance and shortness of breath.[8]

Symptoms of "Aplastic Crisis"

- ✓ Paleness, fever, headache
- ✓ Lethargy or very tired
- ✓ "Not feeling good"
- ✓ Abnormal Yellow eyes or skin
- ✓ Very dark urine
- ✓ Anemia (low blood count)
- ✓ Recent upper respiratory infection
- ✓ Passing out (fainting)

Who is susceptible to Aplastic Crisis?

Children under the age of 16 typically experience Aplastic crisis. It is usually detected in individuals with compromised immune systems, chronic anemia and specifically those with sickle cell disease. Persistent bouts with aplastic crisis are uncommon.

Treatment for Aplastic Crisis

A hospital stay is to be anticipated. Blood transfusion therapy is given until the body starts making red blood cells again. For the most part, hospitalization is required to address this illness.

Is a follow up visit necessary?

Given the nature of this illness, a follow up visit is not an option but an obligation. Following up with your hematologist is important because it identifies changes in health and will enable your doctor to catch any suspected reoccurrences early.

[8] The Comprehensive Sickle Cell Program at Albany Medical Center

Parvovirus B19 or "Fifth Disease"

What You Need to Know

- ✓ Know how to recognize the symptoms

What You Need to Do

- ✓ Be sure the child gets plenty of rest and fluids

What is Parvovirus B19?

Fifth disease (erythema infectiosum) is caused by parvovirus B19. Fifth disease is a mild rash illness that occurs most commonly in children. The ill child typically has a "slapped-cheek" rash on the face and a lacy red rash on the trunk and limbs. Occasionally, the rash may itch. An ill child may have a low-grade fever, malaise, or a "cold" a few days before the rash breaks out. The child is usually not very ill, and the rash resolves in 7 to 10 days.[9]

What causes "fifth disease?"

Fifth disease is caused by infection with human parvovirus B19. This virus infects only humans. Pet dogs or cats may be immunized against "parvovirus," but these are animal parvoviruses that do not infect humans. Therefore, a child cannot "catch" parvovirus from a pet dog or cat, and a pet cat or dog cannot catch human parvovirus B19 from an ill child.[10]

How serious is "fifth disease?"

Parvovirus B19 infection may cause a serious illness in persons with sickle-cell disease. Parvovirus B19 can temporarily slow down or stop the body's production of the oxygen-carrying red blood cells resulting in anemia. Individuals with sickle cell disease are already anemic and can become very sick if the virus further affects their red blood cell production. Their red blood cell levels may drop dangerously low, affecting the supply of oxygen to the body's organs and tissues.

The incubation period (the time between infection and the onset of symptoms) for fifth disease ranges from 4 to 28 days, with the average being 16 to 17 days.[11]

---

[9] http://www.cdc.gov/ncidod/dvrd/revb/respiratory/parvo_b19.htm

[10] http://www.cdc.gov/ncidod/dvrd/revb/respiratory/parvo_b19.htm

[11] http://www.kidshealth.org/parent/infections/skin/fifth.html

Is it Contagious?

Parvovirus B19 spreads from person to person in fluids from the nose, mouth, and throat of someone with the infection, especially through large droplets from coughs and sneezes. It can also be spread through shared drinking glasses and utensils.

There is no vaccine for fifth disease, and no real way to prevent the spread of the virus. Isolating someone with a fifth disease rash won't prevent spread of the infection because the person usually isn't contagious by that time. Practicing good hygiene, especially frequent hand washing, is always a good idea since it can help prevent the spread of infection.[12]

Symptoms of "Fifth Disease"

- ✓ Low grade fever
- ✓ Fatigue
- ✓ Itchy red rash on cheeks
- ✓ Cold like symptoms(cough, runny nose)
- ✓ Red, lace like rash all over body
- ✓ Joint aches and pains

How is Fifth Disease Treated?

Tylenol, hand washing and fluids[13]

Pain Crisis or "Vaso-Occlusive" Crisis

What you need to Know

- ✓ Does your child have a fever with the pain
- ✓ Where the pain is and if it's pain associated with Sickle Cell

[12] http://www.health.state.ny.us/nysdoh/communicable_diseases/en/fifth.htm

[13] http://www.emedicinehealth.com/fifth_disease/page6_em.htm#Fifth%27s%20Disease%20Treatment

- ✓ Level of pain and determine if the pain can be managed at home

What you need to do

Begin treating the pain at home

You will be able to treat the pain according to severity. Your Hematologist will instruct you on how to give Tylenol and/or Ibuprofen. Also, your Hematologist will write a prescription for Tylenol 3 (contains codeine) just to keep at home. If your child's pain is unmanageable at home, get your child to the hospital immediately. **Under no circumstances should you keep the child at home if they are having a rough time.!!!!!!** Remember to call your Hematologist and inform him or her of what is happening. Sometimes you don't have time to call the Hematologist, which is understandable; your child's well-being and instant pain relief comes first.

There is one exception to this- if the child is having pain involving the spleen; my best parental advice is to get the child to the hospital immediately. This crisis can be fatal.

Determine where the pain is

Sickle Cell is very unpredictable. If you are able to, figure out what part of the body is paining your child .

What is a Pain Crisis and What Causes it

A pain crisis is a painful event that can occur in any part of the body as a complication of sickle cell anemia. The exact cause of pain is unknown at this time; however, it is suspected that pain results when sickled cells block small blood vessels thereby preventing the flow of oxygen throughout the body.

Where will the pain occur?

Predicting when a crisis may occur can be difficult. Blockages can occur in any part of the body, although the extremities, chest, stomach, back, feet and bones are commonly affected sites. [14] Painful episodes are not usually dangerous and can last for several hours, days or even up to a week or two.

It is important to be aware of the situations that can trigger a crisis. Dehydration, infection, extreme exercise, alcohol, stress and cold weather are said to be some of the identifying factors known to trigger painful events. Painful events are the most common cause of hospitalizations for sickle cell anemia patients, however, only a small number of individuals with sickle cell experience recurrent and severe painful episodes.

Treating Pain at Home

Painful episodes can be mild, moderate or severe in terms of how much it hurts. Taking over the counter

---

[14] http://www.aafp.org/afp/20000301/1349.html

medication for pain, drinking plenty of liquids and other home remedies usually relieves discomfort. Some over the counter medications that can be used at home are Tylenol (acetaminophen) and Motrin (ibuprofen). Other home remedies include rest, warm baths, and massage, heating pads or electric blankets. If the home remedies are not working, you may need to take Tylenol with codeine. If you do not have a prescription for Tylenol with codeine you will have to contact your physician.
If the pain is so severe where the above remedies will not work, seek medical attention. There may be a need for stronger medications that will be administered in the hospital intravenously.

Pain that is an Emergency

- ✓ Severe Headaches
- ✓ Shortness of breath
- ✓ Stomach pain
- ✓ Pain with fever, swelling and redness .i.e. pain not relieved by home remedies i.e. heating pads, warm baths, massage, Tylenol, Motrin, rest, increased fluids

Hand and Foot Syndrome or "Dactylitis"

What you need to know

- ✓ The symptoms

What you need to do

- ✓ Be able to recognize the symptoms

What is Hand & Foot Syndrome?

When the small blood vessels in the hands and feet are obstructed, pain, swelling and possibly fever may occur. This may be the first symptom of sickle cell anemia in infants and young children. When this occurs the child will not want to walk and will not allow you to touch their hands or feet. One in four infants born with sickle cell disease may experience at least one episode of "hand and foot" syndrome by the age of 2 years old. Hand & foot syndrome generally occurs during the first 3 years of life. An episode may last for 1 or 2 weeks.

Symptoms of Hand & Foot Syndrome

- ✓ Extreme pain and tenderness in hands and feet
- ✓ Fever
- ✓ Tingling and burning sensations
- ✓ Redness
- ✓ Experiences pain when walking

How is hand & foot syndrome treated?

The goal of treatment is to relieve pain, prevent infections, and control complications if they occur. Treatment includes the use of pain medication and fluids.

Acute Chest Syndrome

What you need to know

- ✓ The symptoms

What you need to do

- ✓ Be able to recognize the symptoms

What is Acute Chest Syndrome?

Acute Chest Syndrome (ACS) is a life threatening complication of sickle cell anemia that should be treated in the hospital. This is similar to pneumonia, with symptoms such as difficulty breathing, chest pain and fever. ACS can occur at any age but occurs most commonly in children, however, is more severe in adults. ACS is caused by infection or blocked blood vessels (sickling) in the small blood vessels of the lungs. This complication is similar to pneumonia but is distinct from pneumonia. Individuals affected may experience fever, cough, chest pain and shortness of breath.[15]

Signs of Acute Chest Syndrome

- ✓ Sometimes the chest hurts so bad that the pain spreads to the stomach.
- ✓ Fever of 101°F or 38.5°C or higher.
- ✓ Very congested cough.

[15] http://www.healthatoz.com

- ✓ Troubled and fast breathing.
- ✓ Chest pain
- ✓ You may see your child's ribs "suck in" when he/she breathes in.

How is ACS treated?

There are several types of treatments available for ACS. Treatments may include antibiotics, blood transfusions, pain medications, oxygen and medicines that help open up blood vessels and improve breathing.[16]

Should ACS be treated at home?

No!!!!!!! ACS has the potential to travel from one end of the spectrum to the other real fast and sudden…. **((((((MINOR ↔ SERIOUS))))).** It is therefore recommended that one seek medical attention immediately.

Stroke

What you need to know

- ✓ The symptoms

What you need to do

- ✓ Be able to recognize the symptoms

What is a stroke?

Strokes result in compromised release of oxygen to an area of the brain. The cost of stroke can range from life threatening, to severe physical or cognitive impairments, apparent or subtle learning disabilities to undetectable effects. Less than 1 in 10 individuals with sickle cell anemia will have a stroke.[17]

What causes stroke?

If sickle-shaped cells block a blood vessel in the brain, a stroke can result. This can lead to lasting

[16] http://www.marchofdimes.com/professionals/681_1221.asp

[17] http://www.tdh.state.tx.us/newborn/sickle.htm

disabilities, including learning problems. Doctors can sometimes identify children who are at increased risk of stroke using a special type of ultrasound examination called a "transcranial doppler."[18]

Signs of a Stroke

- ✓ Jerking or twitching of the face, legs, arms.
- ✓ Convulsions or seizures.
- ✓ Strange, abnormal behavior.
- ✓ Inability to move an arm and/or a leg.
- ✓ Staggering or an unsteady walk when your child walked normally before.
- ✓ Stuttered or slurred speech when your child had clear speech before.
- ✓ Weakness in the hands, feet or legs.
- ✓ Changes in vision.
- ✓ Severe headaches that won't go away with Tylenol.
- ✓ Severe vomiting.

Treatment for Stroke

If your child is determined to be at high risk for stroke a doctor may recommend regular blood transfusions to help prevent a stroke from happening.

Gallstones & Jaundice

What you need to know

- ✓ The symptoms of gallstones and Jaundice
- ✓ What is a gallbladder
- ✓ What is its purpose
- ✓ What are gallstones
- ✓ What is Jaundice

What you need to do

- ✓ Be able to recognize the symptoms of a gallbladder attack and/or jaundice

[18] http://health.msn.com/kids-health/articlepage.aspx?cp-documentid=100169868

What is a gallbladder and how does it function?

The gallbladder acts as a link between the liver (which produces bile necessary for the digestion of fats) and the small intestine, where the digestion occurs. The gallbladder stores the bile and releases it as needed.[19]

What is Bile?

Bile is a thick digestive fluid secreted by the liver and stored in the gallbladder. It facilitates digestion by breaking down fats into fatty acids, which can be absorbed by the digestive tract. Bile contains mostly cholesterol, bile acids (also called bile salts), and bilirubin (a breakdown product of hemoglobin). Bile also contains very small amounts of excreted copper and other metals.[20]

Bilirubin?

Bilirubin is a result of the rapid breakdown of the hemoglobin and is the final product of hemoglobin destruction, which is typically removed from the bloodstream by the liver. Due to constant and excessive red blood cell destruction, bilirubin production is increased thereby causing gallstones to form in the gallbladder.

What are gallstones and how are they formed?

Gallstones are pieces of solid material that form in the gallbladder. Gallstones form when substances in the bile, primarily cholesterol and bile pigments, form hard, crystal-like particles. [21] Children with sickle-cell disease have an increased risk for gallstones. About 30% of children with sickle-cell disease have gallstones, and, by age 30, 70% of patients have them. In most cases, gallstones do not cause symptoms for years. When symptoms develop, patients may feel overly full after meals, have pain in the upper right quadrant of the abdomen, or have nausea and vomiting. Acute attacks can be confused with a sickle-cell crisis in the liver. Ultrasound is usually used to confirm a diagnosis of gallstones.[22]

Treatment for Gallstones

If symptoms are not present then treatment may not be necessary. If there is pain from gallstones, the gallbladder may need to be removed. Simple procedures such as laparoscopy reduce possible complications.

---

19 http://www.jcr.org/index.php?module=articles&action=view&ID=17

20 http://www.nlm.nih.gov/medlineplus/ency/article/002237.htm

21 www.gastro.com

22 http://adam.about.com/reports/000058_5.htm

What is Jaundice?

You may notice yellowing in the eyes and/or skin tone. This is known as jaundice and is caused by increasing levels of bilirubin, which occurs as a result of the rapid breakdown of the red blood cells. Therefore, jaundice and an enlarged liver can also be a sign of a poorly functioning liver. Increased bilirubin can also result in a greater chance of gallstones. Treatment may include the removal of the gall bladder and/or gallstones should they cause any symptoms.

Signs of Gallbladder attack

- ✓ Chest pain in the right side (caused by stones in the bile duct or inflammation or swelling of the gallbladder itself)
- ✓ Nausea and/or vomiting
- ✓ Gas, bloating
- ✓ Right side of stomach is very tender to touch
- ✓ Pain traveling through back shoulder blade
- ✓ Constipation

Priapism (specific to the male child)

What you need to know

The symptoms

What you need to do

Be able to recognize the symptoms

What is Priapism?

Priapism is a complication of sickle cell anemia specific to males. This condition is characterized by a constant and painful erection of the penis. Due to blood vessel blockage by sickled cells, blood is trapped in the tissue of the penis. This condition may occur for a brief or extended periods of time. Priapism that occurs for a period longer than 3 hours is characterized as "prolonged" and a period ranging from a few minutes but less than 3 hours is known as "stuttering." Severe episodes often begin during sleep or following sexual activity; but frequently there is no precipitating event or cause. Also, there is no way to predict who will develop priapism or impotence. Because this condition can be extremely painful and can cause damage to the penis tissue resulting in impotence, prompt medical treatment is necessary. Specific causes of priapism are unknown but it is suspected that priapism can be triggered by low oxygen, drinking alcohol or extended periods of sexual intercourse. [23]

Symptoms & Causes

- ✓ Painful erection that will not settle
- ✓ A full bladder can trigger an episode
- ✓ Prolonged sexual activity
- ✓ Alcohol consumption
- ✓ Infection

How is Priapism treated?

The goal of treatment is to ease pain and make the erection go away. Treatment includes hydration, medication, blood transfusion and surgery.

Bedwetting

What you need to know

The symptoms

What you need to do

Be able to recognize the symptoms

Causes of Bedwetting

According to the State of New Jersey's Department of Health, children with sickle cell urinate more frequently because their kidneys do not hold water well. This can result in a child wetting the bed through no fault of his/her own. This may occur until the child realizes that she/he should get up at night to use the bathroom.

What You Should Do

You may also help the child by setting your alarm and waking the child up to use the bathroom. Because the child is not fully awake, I would recommend that you assist the child and see him/her through the process (no matter how old he or she is). I would further suggest you keep a sippy cup (yes , a sippy cup) available at all times (maybe on the nightstand) and encourage the child to drink

[23] http://www.fpnotebook.com/hemeonc/Hemoglobin/PrpsmInScklClAnm.htm

after urinating. This may seem inconvenient but believe me, it is not more inconvenient than spending your nights in the hospital! **Caution: under no circumstances should you give the child less fluid to prevent bed-wetting. It is very important that they remain hydrated at all times.**

Kidney Problems

What you need to know

The symptoms

What you need to do

Be able to recognize the symptoms

Symptoms of Kidney Problems

- ✓ Urinating more than usual
- ✓ Blood in the urine
- ✓ Pain when urinating
- ✓ Wetting the bed

What you should do

As with any major organ, my first advice will always be to contact your child's Hematologist and let him/her know what is going on. When it comes to major organs there is no second guessing! There are suggestions such as treating a kidney issue with medication, but you "must" get the medication from the Hematologist as soon as possible!

End of Chapter Note

I covered a few medical issues that may arise while caring for your child and that must be given immediate attention. I also shared some tips that I learned along the way. The medical issues highlighted in this chapter are far from exhaustive. I further believe it is important to share a few words and phrases that have no place in my vocabulary when it comes to my child's medical care. They include, but are not limited to :

- ✓ "I can't"
- ✓ "I'm tired"
- ✓ "I have to work"

- ✓ "I will take care of that later"
- ✓ "Don't worry about it"
- ✓ "It's not that serious"
- ✓ " I will call the doctor in the morning"
- ✓ "I don't know"

Please eliminate these phrases from your vocabulary too!

Chapter 5

Sickle Cell & Annual Testing

What You Need to Know

"Doppler ultrasound scanning measures blood flowing through the carotid arteries or the arteries at the base of the brain. This test assesses the risk of stroke."[24]

What You Need to do

✓ **Have this test repeated annually.**
Your Hematologist will have the test scheduled for you.

An Experience: The Transcranial Doppler Tech is a Novice!

I bring my child to the clinic for a Transcranial Doppler (TCD) scan annually, (you will do the same with your child). From year to year you will become familiar with the technicians and be able to recognize them. This one particular year the tech that would be performing the scan was a new face to us. However, simply because he was new to us didn't necessarily mean that he was just hired, after all we haven't been there in a year. So we go into the exam room, my child lays on the table, and the tech begins the ultrasound. I notice as he proceeded he seemed really confused and then called in someone else for help. The tech that came to help him has been in that department for years, it was actually our technician from last year. So the tech from last year helps the new guy and leaves. Approximately 60 seconds later the new guy is summoning the tech again. He comes in and helps him once again. This routine repeated itself at least 4 more times within 15 minutes. I was becoming more concerned with each passing moment. The concern must have been written all over my

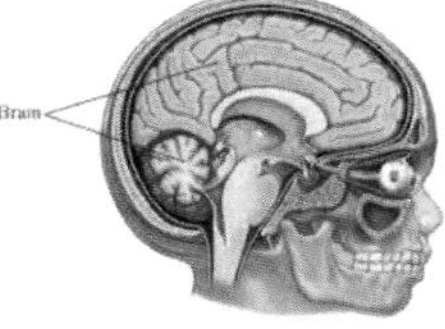

EMPOWHER.COM 1

[24] http://www.csmc.edu/Patients/Programs-and-Services/Neurology/Diagnostic-Services/Transcranial-Doppler.aspx

face because the tech suddenly blurts out, "I have never done one of these tests." Oh my goddddddddddddd, are you kidding me!!!!!!!!!!!! To put it mildly, I was getting pissed by the minute. Not only have we been in this room for almost an hour but there has been no progress. Fueling the fire was the realization that this guy was "practicing" on my child. As you can imagine every curse word known to man began running through my head (I may have even invented a few new ones that day) and I had all I could do to prevent them from spewing out of my mouth. Instead, I checked myself and "requested" that he call the other tech who had helped him earlier.

What is the point of me sharing this? The point is simple, when you bring your child in to have his/her TCD completed, don't be afraid to inquire about the tech's experience with completing this certain test. I was only able to recognize that this guy was practicing on my child and did not know what he was doing because I had this test completed in the past years. If this is your child's first time having the test completed you may not recognize the signs of a novice. Inquiring will save you lots of time, frustration and pisstivity!

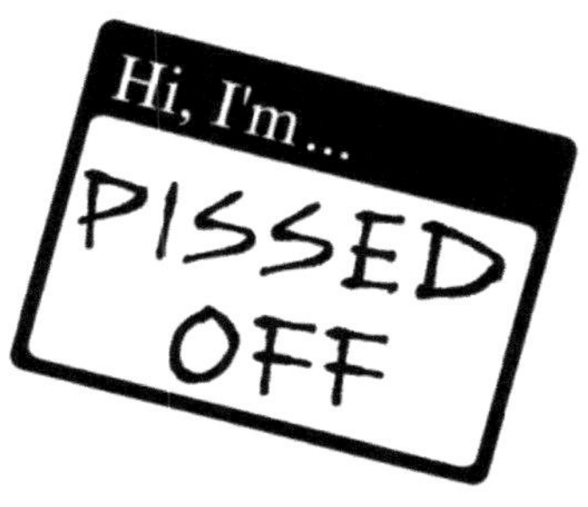

LOVELYBEAUTIFULMESS.BLOGSPOT.COM 1

Chapter 6

Other Things to Be Aware of

The Emergency Room Visit

What you need to know

- ✓ What symptoms necessitated urgent medical care
- ✓ Child's last fever and pain
- ✓ Last time child has taken any medication
- ✓ Your child's past and current treatment course and complications

What you need to do

- ✓ You need to ensure that your child is receiving proper medical care in a timely fashion
- ✓ You need to be active in every aspect of Emergency Room care
- ✓ You need to ask questions when you don't understand the care that is being given to your child

The Emergency Room Visit

Good Lord! The emergency room visit can be a good or bad experience. Yes, you've read right! Unfortunately, not all of your experiences will be pleasant ones when taking your child into the ER. Obviously if you are taking your child to the ER something major is going on like a very high fever, dehydration, vomiting, or "PAIN!" Whatever is going on at the time, it's pretty safe to assume that you're probably in hard-core panic mode. My best advice is to try to remain

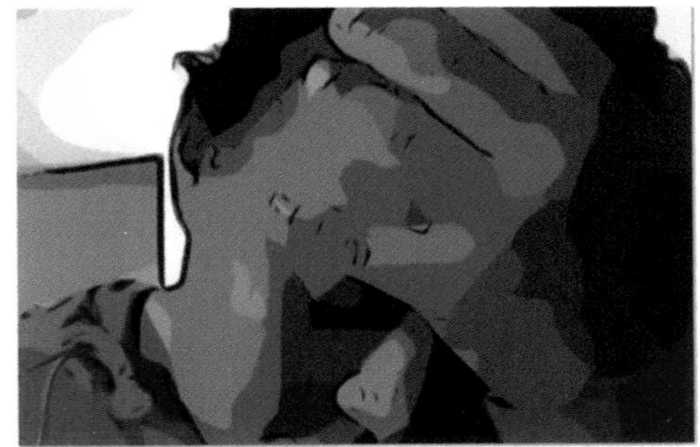

calm and communicate clearly with the hospital staff. Your objective is to inform them of what necessitated this visit, what specifically is going on and how long it's been going on. You will be bombarded with question after question after question. You want to be sure to know what medications the child is prescribed, what specific medications the child took before coming into the ER, when the next dose is due, your child's medical history, last hospitalization, baseline temperatures and health insurance information. Yes, they want to get paid! I know this sounds like a lot and it is, I will show you how to answer all of the questions easily while under stress. Now that we've discussed what is expected of you when you bring the child in, now lets discuss what is expected of your Hematologist and the ER staff.

Upon arrival to the ER there is an expectation of immediate, quality care for your child. Does this always happen? No it doesn't! Please don't be caught off guard, the element of surprise can be baffling to say the least. First things first, the Emergency Room has a standard protocol for treating pediatric sickle cell anemia patients. For instance, if it is fever the child should be treated with antibiotics immediately. If it is pain they will measure the pain, find the source and treat it and so on. Sometimes this does not happen in a timely fashion and if you fail to advocate for your child s/he could fall through the cracks. Falling through the cracks would mean a longggggg waiting period before receiving care. There is no excuse for this. If you placed the call to your Hematologist and your Hematologist gives the emergency room staff a heads up, they should be expecting you and be prepared to act. Will you be their only patient that has an emergency and needs to be seen? No! Does your sickle cell related illness rate high amongst the most important cases? Without a doubt!!! So what do you do if the emergency room is failing to follow their standard protocol? You advocate for your child. You are going to actively communicate your child's needs to the ER staff and that means taking every measure necessary to ensure that your child receives the care s/he needs. (I don't recommend punching anyone's lights out though). Yes there will be times when the frustration becomes unbearable but you **"must"** keep your anger in check. There is nothing worse than a parent that is angry and unable to communicate their child's needs to change the situation; your child will be the one to suffer as a result.

So You Wanna Fight???

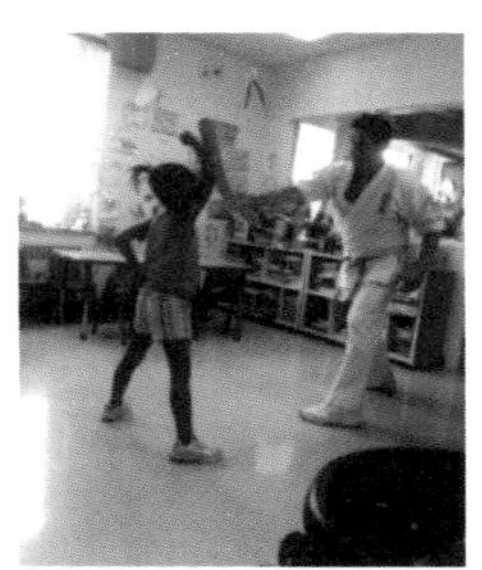

If I have to fight for adequate Medical Treatment for my child, you will fight to keep your State Certified Medical License! No More "Business as Usual!"

While writing this the thought of the situation that I am about to share actually pisses me off all over again. Just recently my child experienced a delay in emergency medical care. I contacted the on-call first to inform them that I was on my way into the ER. We arrived and she continued to vomit and could hold nothing down. My child was violently vomiting. It was apparent that she was dehydrating. We get into the ER and are ushered straight into an exam room.. The RN came in to assess what was going on and to take vitals. After that, we waited over an hour without being seen by a Physician or anyone else for that matter.

I again called the Hematology on-call while I sat in the ER to see if the Hematologist would be able to connect with the attending physician and get my child treated a bit quicker. Within this hour my child had continued to vomit until there was nothing else to vomit. Her eyes were sunken and her lips were pasty. She had become so dehydrated that her veins were disappearing.

So I went out to ask the RN what was going on and explained that my child was dehydrating and on the hills of a pain crisis. The RN tells me that they had forty-two other patients in the ER and that my child was not the only patient." I felt my blood boil; it felt like hot lava running through my veins.

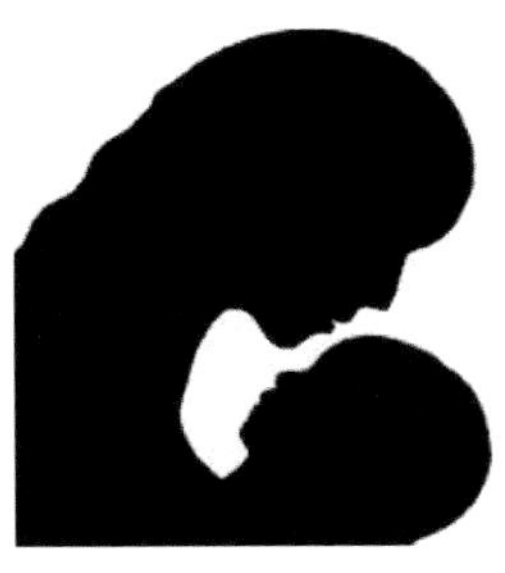

CHRISTFREE.COM 1

I then asked the RN where the attending physician was and requested to see him. The nurse then immediately came back with, "he's busy right now!" I then asked what his name was. The RN would not provide his name. I then told the RN that it was too easy to find out who he is by contacting the Human Resource office in the morning. I further informed the RN that there is a standard protocol that must be followed when treating a child with Sickle Cell. The RN then responded, "we get them all the time." So I told him that he had the right person today because tomorrow morning I would be contacting the hospitals patient relations, the New York State Office of Professional Medical Conduct and Physician Discipline and the **Joint Commission on Accreditation of Healthcare Organizations (JCAHO)**. I told him that he could pass the information on to the "unnamed" attending physician. He walked out and in about a hot 60 seconds the RN comes back and starts my child's IV(he could have got the order far much earlier since the prevailing condition reported was sickle cell and vomiting).

The RN then goes on to ask if I wanted morphine for my child, this was without examining her nor seeing a doctor. I then asked how did the doctor determine that morphine was needed without seeing my child. The RN said the doctor looked at her chart and wrote a script for it already. Really? Finally the attending physician comes in and apologizes and thanks me for my patience. I am thinking, "please spare me!" I hate to feel this angry and to hold such a level of hostility against medical professionals that are supposed to be treating my child. This is only one of a few incidents that has caused me to adopt the *"If I have to fight for adequate medical treatment for my child, you will fight to keep your State Certified Medical License"* attitude. It seems that some medical professionals only understand you when their State license and livelihood becomes endangered. I hope no one reading this book ever experiences a situation like this. If there is one lesson to be learned it is that you must not tolerate the "business as usual" attitudes or inaction on the part of medical staff when bringing your child to the ER .

The Hospital Admission aka Overnight Stay

What you need to know

- ✓ Your child's medical history
- ✓ Your child's current medications
- ✓ You "should not' leave your child in the hospital overnight alone

What do you need to do

- ✓ *Assemble your support network (people that can rotate with you during your child's stay)*

At some point your child will have to be admitted into the hospital. Always anticipate that your child will be staying for a minimum of 3 days. You're going to need a support network. Your support network should include people that are willing and able to rotate and stay in the hospital with your child when admitted. This will allow you time to take care of things and be assured that your child is not alone. You may be thinking that there is hospital staff there always and this is true. I would not advise any parent to leave their child in the hospital alone overnight with only staff to attend to the child's needs. This is a major "NO, NO!" Just be aware that each nurse is assigned a certain number of patients who also have pressing needs. Just think, your child's IV machine may be beeping, your child may need help to go to the bathroom (while hooked up to the IV pole), your child may be hungry, your child may not be able to reach his/her remote or call button and your child may be faced with a stranger standing at the foot of the bed ready to draw blood . These are all very real situations that arise during a hospital admission. Your child will need someone representing and helping them at all times.

- ✓ ***Keep a reserve of cash that you will use "only" when your child is admitted***
  Don't get caught out there broke!!!!!!!
  You should also keep a reserve of extra cash. Remember it is not a matter of "If" your child will be admitted but "when!" While your child is hospitalized the show must go on at home. The bills will continue to roll in. Nothing stops because your child is ill and admitted in the hospital. Take a proactive approach and save a few dollars every week if possible.
- ✓ ***Plan for hospital admissions, keep your home in order and assemble a plan B for the care of your other children (if you have more than one child)***
  If you have other children at home, it is important to have a plan B in place during the time your child has to be hospitalized . You should have someone with whom you can drop your other child(ren) off and be confident that they will be ok.

The 411 on Hospital Admissions

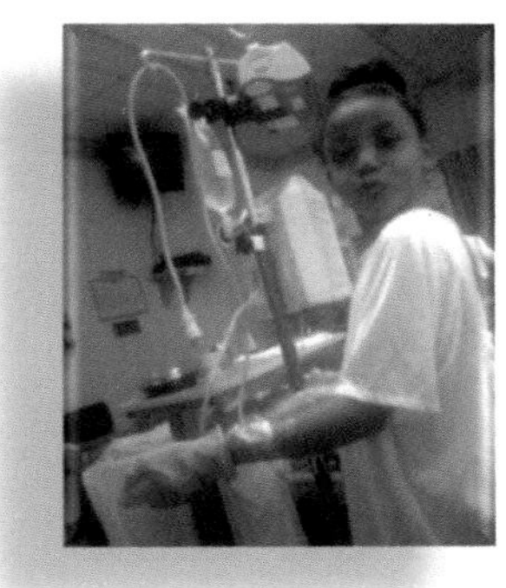

As I said, it is not a matter of "if "your child will be hospitalized, but "when!" To think of your child being hospitalized is frightening. Who wants to see their child all hooked up to IV's or having a blood transfusion? Well this is the reality for us. We must make the most of the hospital stay. Depending on where your child goes for care will make the difference. As I mentioned, my child attends a clinic with patients predominantly being treated for Cancer and Leukemia . It appears that they have lots of funding and the clinic has an amazing set up. If you did not know what the place was ahead of time, one would think that it was a play center. This clinic and pediatric wing reminds you of a Jeepers or Chuck E. Cheese type of setting. It is huge and has everything a child would desire such as the latest game systems, computers, new toys, fish tanks, karate lessons while you wait, a miniature children's library, arts & crafts and a toy room for the patients. You're probably wondering what this has to do with the hospital stay. It's very simple; the atmosphere of the clinic is carried over to the wing of the hospital where the children stay, it has the clinic amenities and a warm homely feeling. The hospital wing has an amazing playroom and a kitchen. Across from the wing is a Ronald McDonald house where there is yet another playroom, kitchen with food provided by volunteers and restaurants, computers, miniature living room and a teen entertainment room. The pediatric wing sort of feels like a "home away from home!" It is so cozy at one point my child was going into crisis and stated, "oh goodie, I get to play." Well if I had to choose I would not want her to be sick but it is comforting that she is ok with going there. Let's face it, she would have to go when

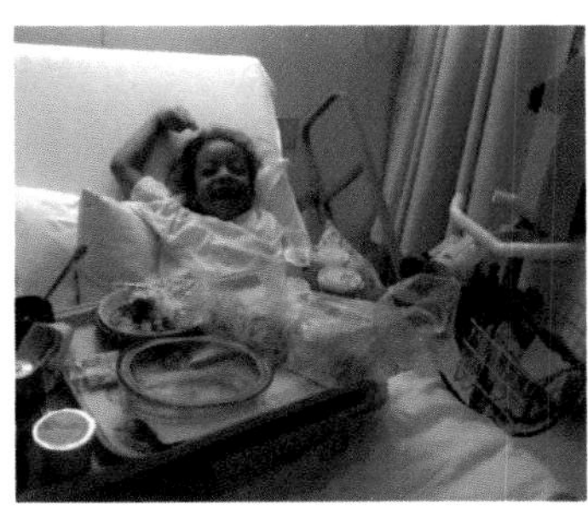

sickle cell says she has to anyway, so it may as well have some level of comfort. I am not saying that you will find this type of atmosphere in every clinic or pediatric hospital wing. I can only tell you what we have experienced. My account may give you an idea of what to expect or have something to compare to. With saying all of that, let's not lose sight of the stay itself. I don't leave my child there alone. I have not turned a blind eye to the shortage of nurses. The nurses have heavy caseloads, call button wait times can be long and I must monitor my child's care every step of the way. Sometimes the hospital staff are more attentive when they are aware that the parent is present.

Chronic Illness, School Policies & the Difference between Individual Education Plans (IEP) and the 504 Accommodations Plan

What You Need to Know

- ✓ School Districts Policy regarding the continuous education of "chronically ill" children
- ✓ Know the difference between a 504 Plan and the IEP
- ✓ Always remember, "If it is not written it didn't happen"—never ever take anyone's word, get it in writing!!!!!!!

What You Need to do

- ✓ ***Schedule a meeting via conference and/or conference call between all parties involved with your child's education***

  When your child becomes school aged you must take a proactive stance and get your child's plan in order before s/he becomes ill. I learned this the hard way by not preparing ahead of time. This is very important because you may face a bit of resistance due to ignorance of the disease or the almighty "budget constraints." To put a plan in place is free, it is what is included in the plan that may become costly for the school district. The goal is to get all the information on your child out there so that everyone is on the same page. You want everyone to know the who, what, when, where and why about your child's chronic illness. Those in attendance should include, but are not limited to, the school nurse, the Special Education Committee Representative, your child's teacher, the principal, your child's Hematologist and Sickle Cell Nurse and anyone involved in the child's care at home.

Request that your child have a 504 and/or IEP Plan in place

The difference between the 504 Accommodations Plan and the IEP Plan follows:

"Section 504 of the Rehabilitation Act guarantees an appropriate special education as well as accessibility to regular education programs. It requires that all children with disabilities be provided a free, appropriate public education in the least restrictive environment. A person with a disability

under Section 504 is any person who (i) has a physical or mental impairment which substantially limits one or more major life activities, (ii) has a record of such an impairment, or (iii) is regarded as having such an impairment."[25]

"The IEP is the cornerstone for the education of a child with a disability. It should identify the services a child needs so that he/she may grow and learn during the school year. It is also a legal document that outlines:

- The child's special education plan by defining goals for the school year
- Services needed to help the child meet those goals
- A method of evaluating the student's progress

The objectives, goals and selected services are not just a collection of ideas on how the school may educate a child; the school district must educate your child in accordance with the IEP."[26]

✓ ***Keep everyone on the same page***
Everyone involved in your child's care needs to be on the same page for reason such as accountability, clarity and to alleviate confusion. Having a chronic illness is very serious and there is zero room for mistakes (mistakes can be prevented). Keep in mind that you may be the primary caretaker of your child so you must plan for the worse. Tomorrow is not promised to any of us. If something were to happen to you, you would want someone to be able to step in and take over, thereby ensuring continued care for your child. You want that person to be able to hit the ground running.

✓ ***Some Requests you may consider for your 504 or IEP Plan***
Request that your child be given bathroom breaks "as needed," request that your child be placed on a drinking schedule and be monitored (You provide the fluid) , request that your child not be forced to participate in outside recess in extreme hot or cold temperatures, request temperatures, request tutoring whenever child is hospitalized, (you will probably need your Hematologist write a letter on your behalf regarding this issue)

School Administration and Teachers Must Understand the Child diagnosed Sickle Cell Disease

It is important that school administration and teachers understand sickle cell disease, the health concerns of the child, and associated risks for the child. The goal is for the child to actively participate in a regular school setting, however, there is still the risk of the child having complications while in school. These complications cannot go untreated and school officials must be ready to act. Most likely the child will need or already have a 504 accommodations plan or an IEP in place, which should provide specific instructions regarding the child's medical care in the event of a complication.

---

[25] http://www.ed-center.com/504

[26] http://www.autism-society.org/site/PageServer?pagename=life_edu_IEP

Because having a sickle cell crisis is very unpredictable, school staff should always expect the unexpected.

My Best Advice to You….

I hesitated about writing this , but it is needed. Be ready to battle your school district. I didn't say that you should start the battle, but be ready! There is always a possibility that an issue may arise, particularly while trying to obtain tutoring services for your child as soon as he or she is hospitalized. Some school districts will lead you to believe that the district is in complete control. Wrong! I told you that you are your child's best advocate and it is you that will be monumental in planning for your child's educational needs and when creating your child's educational plan (504 or IEP). Never lose sight of the fact that school districts are always looking to cut cost. I will even go a step further and tell you that they rely on your ignorance of the federal and state educational laws that are in place to ensure your child's receives his or her special educational needs. You must become very familiar with these laws (Family Educational Rights and Privacy Act [FERPA] and Individuals with Disability Education Act [IDEA]) and become fluent. Your knowledge is key when attending any meeting with school administration to discuss your child's special education needs. When these meetings are planned, you will be informed that you have the option to have a "parent advocate" present at the meeting. Don't be blindsided by the "parent advocate" crap as I was told by an attorney. The parent advocate is not your personal advocate. The parent advocate is a parent of a child with special needs (does not necessarily mean their child has the same diagnosis as yours). As with various medical diagnosis', educational needs will vary. The parent advocate will sit in the meeting, and in my experience, they haven't advocated for anything on behalf of my child. I found that reading federal and state laws regarding special education, bringing a tape recorder to every meeting and knowing all about due process were the tools of advocacy that I needed. I strongly urge you to bring an audio recorder to every meeting (and the law says you can). This will allow you to keep a record of what was discussed and also provides an opportunity for you to go back and listen to it as many times as you need to.

Pharmacy and Medication Insurance Coverage

What you need to know

- ✓ You need to know the Pharmacy's operating hours
- ✓ Refill policy
- ✓ If your medical coverage is accepted for the prescriptions you need to fill
- ✓ If the pharmacy accepts supplemental medication coverage plans
- ✓ Are you enrolled in any discount programs offered by this pharmacy

What you need to do

- ✓ ***Be sure your medical insurance is current***
  Always be sure that your medical coverage is up to date because your child will always have prescriptions to fill. The last thing a mother wants to hear from the Pharmacist is that the medical coverage is not active. Those are like fighting words!
- ✓ ***Be sure to call in your scripts well in advance***
  Always call your scripts in early to assure refills as needed.
- ✓ ***Be sure that your scripts are ready before you actually go to the pharmacy for pickup***
  Once your scripts are called in, you may be given an estimated time to pick the scripts up. Please call ahead of time to ensure that the scripts are ready to go. You must account for delayed orders to the Pharmacy, weather conditions, human error, scripts not written right or not legible, short staff, lunch hours and any thing else you can think of. It is just easier to call and confirm that your scripts are ready to go! If you have a special order, call way ahead of time (days before). An example of special orders can include chemotherapy medications (hydroxurea) or pull-ups (the drug store usually carries a limited quantity).

Pharmacy and Insurance Coverage, Arggg!!!!!

You child will need several medications on a consistent basis so filling prescriptions will become a normal part of life for you and your child. Your child can be prescribed several medications or just one medication, regardless, this script will need to be filled on a consistent basis (as prescribed). My best advice for you when dealing with the pharmacy is the following:

IPHARMD.NET 1

1. Please be sure that your child's insurance information remains updated at all times. If your child has a secondary insurance plan be sure to update that as well. It would be best to know about the insurance plan(s) and what your prescription plan allows and what your plan does not cover. Your child needs his/her medication so you don't want to be caught off guard.
2. If there is a co-pay on the first prescription plan and the second plan covers this, please be sure that your pharmacist is clear on this.
3. Be sure to stay up to date with any changes in your medical coverage, especially co-pays.
4. Be sure that your prescriptions and refills are up to date. This is easy to do these days because hospitals and pharmacies are collaborating and using electronic scripts. When you run out of a medication you let your pharmacist know and s/he will contact your physicians office and in return will receive an electronic prescription. **(((PLEASE KNOW)))** that this electronic method will not be used for controlled substances. You must show your identification at the doctor's office and pick up the script. You then take the script to the pharmacy and they will fill it, however, you must have your state identification that includes your picture, to pick up the medication.
5. To avoid potential issues, mixups, miscommunications or whatever you want to call it-call the pharmacy before going to pick up your medication. If you are catching the bus calling will

prove to be more beneficial. Just because you order the refill doesn't always mean it will be there on time. Things happen!

6. As with any medical professional involved with your child's care in some way (pharmacist, specialist, dental, PCP, Social Worker) always be sure to keep a clear and open line of communication!

A Parent's Asset- Forming Healthy Relationships

What you need to know

- ✓ The role of each physician on your child's medical team

What you need to do

- ✓ Form healthy, positive parent-provider relationships with all hospital staff involved in your child's life
- ✓ Be sure that you remain compliant with your child's medical treatment

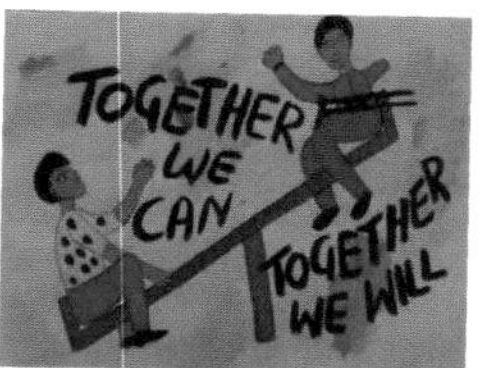

DISABILITYINDIA.COM

Positive relationships with your child's medical providers can yield very positive result driven medical care. Have you ever heard the old cliché, "you get more with sugar than vinegar?" Well that holds true in any situation. An important facet of health care is building and maintaining positive relationships between you and your child's doctors. Fostering a positive relationship with all of our child's doctors can result in quality healthcare. If you're able to communicate well with each other, your child's needs will not only be met but will be met with excellence. In no way am I insinuating that treatment will be substandard if there isn't a positive relationship, however, forming a positive relationship makes the medical experience much more pleasant and much less frustrating.

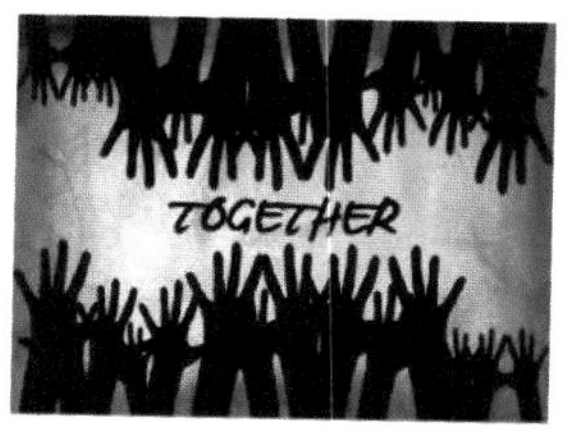

CHADCOTTLE.WORDPRESS.COM

When managing sickle cell disease the Hematologist will be involved in your family's life indefinitely. You and your Hematologist will know one another by name and he/she should be comfortable when communicating with the family. You in turn should feel at ease when communicating with the Hematologist, and all doctors, caring for your child. The Hematologist will also know if your family is compliant with the prescribed treatment plan and will also be familiar with the family's limits and expectations. Going back to our discussion about a team of doctors working with your child, just remember that it would be wise to form a positive parent-provider relationship with each and every one. Will they all treat your child? Maybe! The clinic my child attends has 5 Hematologists on staff and they all know her and are familiar with her course of care. You must also always be prepared for those times when your main doctor is absent due to illness, was promoted to a new position or simply has gone on vacation (they're allowed you know). If this happens you won't slip into panic mode because the other members of the team know your child and can pick up where the other left off without missing a beat.

Combating Preconceived Notions

This type of thinking may amaze you but if you're anything like me, nothing will amaze you. Let's examine my first point and why I hold such an opinion. When I state medical professionals believe that parent's of children diagnosed with sickle cell are not really involved in their child's care, I am referring to the "set ideas" held by some doctors that treat our children. In the beginning, when I brought my child in for treatment I sometimes encountered the "*ok, you got the child to us and everything else is up to us*" mentality. With this type of attitude you will find that all you will get from them is a bunch of questions; however, when it comes to the course of treatment, they decide what they are going to do without explaining what their course of treatment is going to be and why. I have encountered some residents and veteran doctors that just began to act on their course of treatment (during hospitalization); walk past me as if I were invisible, my child laid out on the bed, and began treating her as if she were there alone. Personally, I did not stand for this arrogant behavior and have been very vocal about it whenever confronted with it. If I am there with my child it is only right that the treating physician explain to me what is going on, including an explanation regarding any course of treatment they propose. If there is an instance where my child is terminal, by all means, proceed as needed. This would be my only exception.

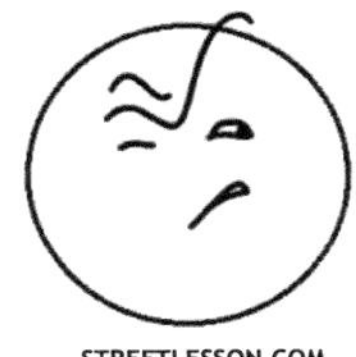
STREETLESSON.COM

Secondly, when I say that there are "set ideas" amongst some of the medical practitioners which may include the belief that we parents are unable to comprehend what is going on with our child's treatment and we are not interested in learning. It seems that they have this notion that we have our heads stuck in the sand. Depending on where you live in the nation (North or South) some of this stereotypical treatment lingers. There seems to be a lack of cultural competence amongst the medical community. Further, there seems to be a belief that the only part of this disease that we understand is the concept of pain and morphine. Wrong! Of course, morphine sometimes is required in the treatment of our child , however, this is not all we are able to understand. If I am able to pick up a book and read, I am able to comprehend. If for some reason I am confused about the information that I am reading, I am going to ask questions, many questions, until I understand. I will ask for a hooked-on-phonics version if I have to. There is no shame in my game! This is my child and I do what I have to do to stay informed and learn about her disease and treatment.

A System of Checks & Balances: Know How to File a Complaint

Hopefully you will not need to use this section, but there is always "one" that will bring you to this section of the book!"

What You Need to Know

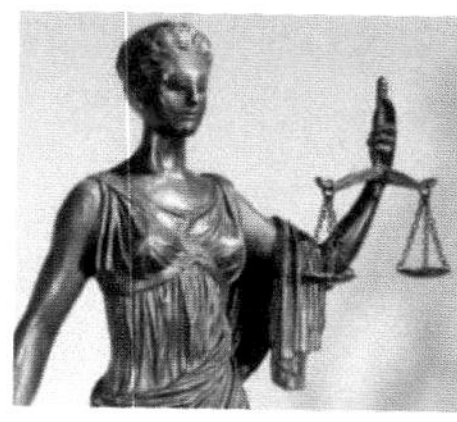

CANCERCOMPASS.COM

- ✓ The issue at hand
- ✓ The procedure for filing a grievance
- ✓ How to navigate the chain of command internally and what options are available externally
- ✓ Know what your options are for filing external complaints

What You Need to do

- ✓ If you are perplexed about the medical care your child is receiving I would suggest you do the following:
    1. Talk to the Physician about your concerns
    2. Ask questions if you do not understand something
    3. Realize that the situation can be a misunderstanding between both parties

Once you have attempted to solve a situation and you are still not satisfied with the answers given or the outcome, you then have a few choices. You can file a complaint internally, externally, or both. My best advice is to try to resolve it first; the outcome may surprise you. If your concerns fall on deaf ears, you can do the following:

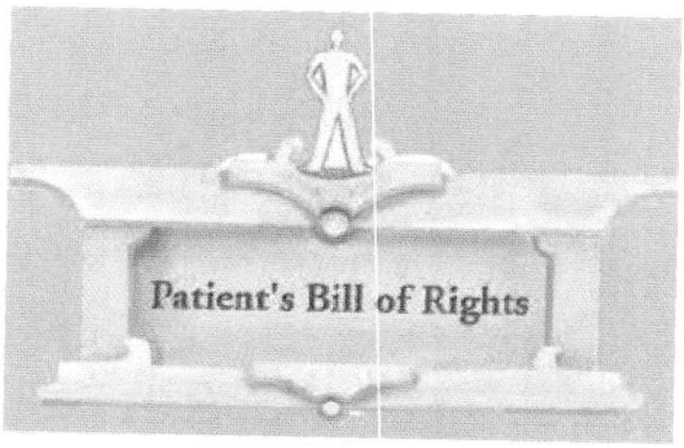

Patient's Bill of Rights

ONEWORLDSEE.ORG

Internally

- ✓ Call the main number of the hospital or clinic and ask for the "patient relations" office of the hospital or clinic in question
- ✓ Once you've contacted that office, explain your situation and ask what the process is for filing a complaint. Whatever the process is follow it and submit your complaint.
- ✓ Once you've reached the right person via phone or face-to-face, they may ask you to explain what is going on and once you conclude they may tell you that they will look into the matter.

That's great that they are going to do that, however, be sure to submit a written complaint also. Again, be specific about knowing the "written" complaint process and specify that you will be following up with a written version of your account. If that process includes emailing your complaint, be sure to copy yourself on the email. Always remember, in the business world - **"If it isn't written, it didn't happen!"**

Externally

- ✓ Locate your local State Office of Professional Medical Conduct.
- ✓ Inquire about their process, they will definitely ask you to submit your complaint in writing.
- ✓ When you prepare your complaint be sure to communicate your ideas clearly and review your complaint over and over for factual and grammatical errors. Realize that if your issue rises to this level you want to be accurate on all accounts of the situation—the Physician's medical license is on the line and the last thing you want to do is make a mistake in your complaint, this is their livelihood.
- ✓ Wait for a decision from the Office of Professional Medical Conduct.

Reportable Complaints & Incidents According to The New York State Health Department

If you feel that your doctor has practiced negligently or incompetently, or has engaged in illegal or unethical practices, he/she may have committed professional misconduct, and should be reported.

Physicians may be charged with misconduct for:

- ✓ Being impaired by alcohol, drugs, physical or mental disability.
- ✓ Abandoning or neglecting a patient in need of immediate care.
- ✓ Promoting the sale of services, goods, appliances, or drugs in a manner that exploits the patient.
- ✓ Refusing to provide medical care due to race, creed, color, or national origin.
- ✓ Guaranteeing a cure.
- ✓ Performing professional services not authorized by the patient.
- ✓ Willfully harassing, abusing or intimidating a patient.
- ✓ Ordering excessive tests or treatments.
- ✓ Failing to make patient records and X rays available to the patient or another physician on request.
- ✓ Permitting unlicensed persons to perform activities which require a license.
- ✓ Practicing the profession with a suspended or inactive license.

- ✓ Revealing personally identifiable facts, data or information without consent of the patient, except as authorized or required by law.[27]

Reports against physicians, physician's assistant, or a specialist assistant should be submitted in writing and should be mailed to the following:

New York State Department of Health
Office of Professional Medical Conduct
433 River Street, Suite 303
Troy, New York 12180- 2299

Complaints against dentists, nurses, chiropractors, podiatrists, optometrists and psychologists should be submitted in writing and mailed to:

Office of Professional Discipline
NYS Education Department
475 Park Ave. South, 2nd Floor
New York, NY 10016-6901

To complain about service or treatment by a professional licensed to practice by the State of New York, or about illegal practice of a profession by an unlicensed person, complete a COMPLAINT form and send it to the Office of Professional Discipline. Please note, this information is specific to New York State complaints. If you are not located in New York State, you can easily use the internet to find the office in your State. Google the following: "your state" + professional misconduct enforcement.

You may print this form located at http://www.op.nysed.gov/documents/opd-complaint.pdf and fax it to: 212-951-6537. You may also call the Complaint Hotline 1-800-442-8106 or email conduct@mail.nysed.gov.

Submitting Complaints against Health Care Organizations

You must submit new complaints to the address and/or email below. If there is an update after submitting your first complaint, you will also submit to the same.

---

27 http://www.health.state.ny.us/publications/1444/

The Joint Commission (This is a National Organization, covering the United States)
E-Mail: complaint@jointcommission.org
Fax: Office of Quality Monitoring (630) 792-5636
Mail:
Office of Quality Monitoring
The Joint Commission
One Renaissance Boulevard
Oakbrook Terrace, IL 60181
If you have questions about how to file your complaint, you may contact the Joint Commission at this toll free U.S. telephone number, 8:30 to 5 p.m., Central Time, weekdays.(800) 994-6610

HIPPA Violations

The Health Insurance Portability and Accountability Act (HIPAA) is also known as the Kennedy-Kassebaum bill. The Health Insurance Portability and Accountability Act (HIPAA) was passed by Congress in 1996 to set a national standard for electronic transfers of health data. At the same time, Congress saw the need to address growing public concern about privacy and security of personal health data.[28] HIPAA sets a national standard for accessing and handling medical information. Before HIPAA, your right to privacy of health information varied depending on what state you live in. Now, health care providers, health plans and other health care services that operate in all states have to abide by the minimum standards set by HIPAA.
"If you believe that a person, agency or organization covered under the HIPAA Privacy Rule ("a covered entity") violated your (or someone else's) health information privacy rights or committed another violation of the Privacy Rule, you may file a complaint with the Office for Civil Rights (OCR). OCR has authority to receive and investigate complaints against covered entities related to the Privacy Rule. A covered entity is a health plan, health care clearinghouse, and any health care provider who conducts certain health care transactions electronically. Complaints to the Office for Civil Rights must: (1) Be filed in writing, either on paper or electronically; (2) name the entity that is the subject of the complaint and describe the acts or omissions believed to be in violation of the applicable requirements of the Privacy Rule; and (3) be filed within 180 days of when you knew that the act or omission complained of occurred. OCR may extend the 180-day period if you can show "good cause." Any alleged violation must have occurred on or after April 14, 2003 (on or after April 14, 2004 for small health plans), for OCR to have authority to investigate.

Anyone can file written complaints with OCR by mail, fax, or email. If you need help filing a complaint or have a question about the complaint form, please call this OCR toll free number: 1-800-368-1019."

You can submit your complaint in any written format. Include the following in your complaint:

---

28 http://www.privacyrights.org/fs/fs8a-hipaa.htm

- ✓ Your name, full address, home and work telephone numbers, email address.
- ✓ If you are filing a complaint on someone's behalf, also provide the name of the person on whose behalf you are filing.
- ✓ Name, full address and phone of the person, agency or organization you believe violated your (or someone else's) health information privacy rights or committed another violation of the Privacy Rule.
- ✓ Briefly describe what happened. How, why, and when do believe your (or someone else's) health information privacy rights were violated, or how the Privacy Rule otherwise was violated?
- ✓ Any other relevant information.
- ✓ Please sign your name and date your letter.[29]

Tips for Submitting Complaints

- ✓ Always remember, if the complaint isn't written, it didn't happen. Yes, you can verbally complain but in most instances it will not go a long way. When submitting a written complaint, you are essentially creating a paper trail. The complaint must be given the proper attention. Further, if you are not confident that your written complaint will be given the proper attention on the lower level , I would suggest that you copy the person's entire chain of command, thereby, you are not skipping the command but informing the higher ups of what is going on. Chain of command consists of a continuous chain of persons with authority, thus ending at the most senior person. For example, Office Manager ~Senior Manager ~Director~ and so on…until you get to the top person which usually ends at the Chief Executive Officer of the business.
- ✓ If you choose to email the complaint, always copy yourself on the email. This becomes your electronic record and your proof of the complaint.

Record Keeping! Record Keeping! Did I say Record Keeping?

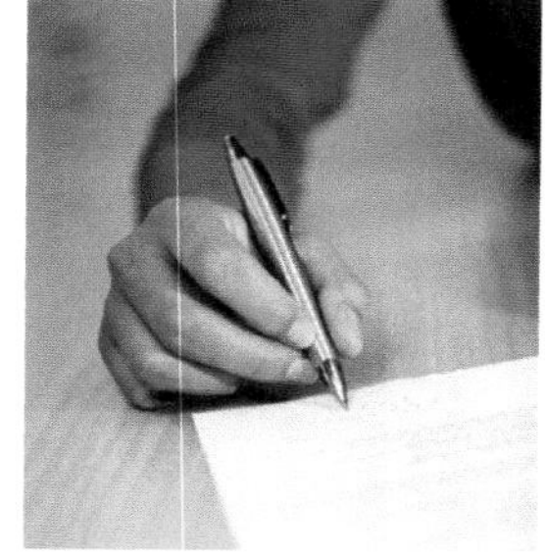
CARL1ANDERSON.WORDPRESS.COM

The digital age has taken record keeping to a new level! In today's world it is very easy to keep track of your child's medical progress and all communications between yourself and your child's medical providers. Once your Pediatrician notifies you that your child has been diagnosed with sickle cell, you're likely to find yourself overcome with shock and disbelief. You are also likely to find yourself walking around in a fog for several days or even weeks. That is the last thing you can afford to let happen. Up to this point my bet is that no one has explained to you the importance of record

[29] http://www.hipaa.ihs.gov/index.cfm?module=faq

keeping. And if they have you may not have "heard" them because you are still in the process of absorbing the news of the diagnosis. Failing to keep records, or getting a late start at doing so, can spell disaster for your child's long term care. When it happens very late there is a lot of missed valuable information that could have and should have been recorded. When taking care of a child with sickle cell please know and expect frequent visits to the hospital or clinic for outpatient and inpatient care. Also be aware that it is possible that your child will be treated by other specialties such as dental, pulmonologist or cardiologist. It is imperative that you record every single bit of information regarding all encounters with the medical team. As I mentioned, when talking about the Emergency Room treatment, there is nothing worse or more aggravating than a doctor asking a bunch of questions when your child is in need, when your patience has worn thin and your stress level is off the charts! To avoid all of the future headaches and the possibility of not knowing when your child received treatment X-Y or Z, it is important to have this information handy. The information you will always need and should document is as follows:

When – when did the symptoms begin, when meaning the date of the current visit and each encounter thereafter

How- how have you treated the symptoms? How did the current symptoms begin?

What-what is currently going on? What is in your child's overall record? Is the current issue new or chronic?

Why-why do you believe your child began to have the current symptoms?

Where-where was the child when the current symptoms began (home, playground, school) ?

It probably seems that the 5 questions are overlapping because they are. This will assist you in preparing and knowing the information to answer every question that you may be asked. Now here is a list of some things you may want to have handy during the visit and after the visit , or while on a trip to the Emergency Room.

1. *Pen & Paper*-I encourage you to keep this in your purse or with you at all times.
2. *Dates*- Document all dates in which your child is seen by "any" medical professional. Something minimal now may mean something big later. Know the date of the visit.
3. *Names of Emergency Room Personnel*- Document all names and titles of all people treating your child in the ER. If this is a routine visit to the Hematologist, document which Hematologist your child saw.
4. *Presenting Symptoms & Treatment Received*- this is going to be key every visit.
5. *Communicate with Treating Professional*- what are they doing to your child and why? Who ordered it? What is the outcome of the procedure or medication in question? Do you agree with the proposed course of treatment?

6. *CBC*-during routine and ER visits your child should have his/her Complete Blood Count drawn. Be sure to ask for a copy of the results of this test. This will be added to your journal.
7. *Review Discharge Forms with Physician*-be sure that the discharge forms reflect the current diagnosis, the reason for the stay and discharge instructions.
8. *Obtain a Copy of Your Child's Medical Records*-write a request for the record in question. You must include your child's name, date of birth, address, date of service and specify where you want the records mailed to. Be sure to sign the request, your request will be denied without a signature.

Documenting your child's medical history will be a lifelong task. I have been documenting everything regarding my child's treatment since she was a few months old. I was advised by the best. Consistently documenting everything has led to expedient and greater quality of care for my child.

The Handicap Permit

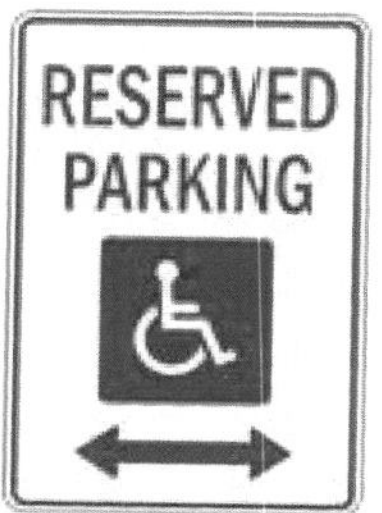

PROPERTYMANAGEMENTSHOP.COM 1

Getting your Hematologist to fill out a form that will allow you to get a handicap permit for your vehicle may be a challenge. Again it will depend on the Hematologist. I asked my child's Hematologist to fill out a form for the permit and she pretty much said that she needed to look into it. What the hell are you looking in to? The Hematologist knows her diagnosis and all about the disease so what's the problem. To make a long story short she said that she would be looking into it and never got back to me. I again asked and again I was ignored. The straw that broke the camel's back was when I had to walk my child from the parking lot to the Emergency Room while the entire time my child was vomiting and rapidly dehydrating. After this experience I asked the Hematologist once more and again received no response regarding this permit. So, taking the "BULL" by the horns, I obtained the actual handicap permit form from the Department of Motor Vehicle and wrote a letter to my child's Primary Care Physician outlining how I had to walk my child to the Emergency Room when she was severely dehydrated and vomiting. I also had to reiterate what her diagnosis was and why I felt that the permit was necessary. (Yes the Primary Care Physician had to be reminded because she doesn't see my child all the time like Hematology does) I left the form and my letter with my fingers crossed. I received the form back in about 2 weeks granting me the permanent handicap permit. Talk about relieved!

Looking back I believe the Hematologist thought that I wanted to obtain the Handicap Permit for my personal benefit. I have no confirmation of this but these are my thoughts. My thing is, I walk 3-6 miles a day, would I really want to use a Handicap permit for myself? A few steps from a parking lot will not kill me if the 3-6 miles doesn't! Go figure!

My child was 7 years old at the time which means we had spent 7 years walking from the parking lot to our destination inside the hospital. My asking for a handicap permit had nothing to do with my benefit but everything to do with my child's well-being.

Advocating 101

What you need to know

- ✓ Never let them see you sweat!

What you need to do

- ✓ *Learn how to advocate for your child*
  The best way to learn how to advocate is trial and error. Hopefully my tips will prevent the error part for you!
- ✓ *Be empowered and stay focused*
  There will be a time when you experience setbacks. Don't be discouraged. Brush your shoulders off and keep moving forward. Moving forward includes going and researching your specified "need, " then deciding what your next move will be. Remember, without struggle there will be no progress![30]
- ✓ *Sharpen your communication skills (verbal and written)*
  Be kind and specify your wants, needs and goals clearly. If this means you must write them out and practice reading off the paper then so be it! There is nothing worse than a parent that is angry and unable to communicate their needs to change the situation; your child will be the one to suffer as a result.
- ✓ *Defuse tension by Listening instead of Reacting*
  Avoid having emotional knee-jerk reactions. There will be a time when some professional involved in your child's life will absolutely get under your skin. Keep cool and calm while controlling your emotions. This is easier said than done, it takes practice. You will hold the power by listening instead of reacting.
- ✓ *Develop Working Relationships with Professionals involved in your child's life*
  Always be respectful. Be open and honest about your concerns. Agree to disagree. You will not like everything that goes on and sometimes you must take the highroad and be the better person. There is no room for competing egos in your child's care.
- ✓ *Research! Research! Research!*
  Research your request. Is it reasonable? Be prepared to answer the "who, what, when, where

[30] Federick Douglas coined this phrase

and why" of your request. This is all a part of defending your request and substantiating the need.

Super Mom!!!!!!!!!! You Are Your Child's Best Advocate!!!!!

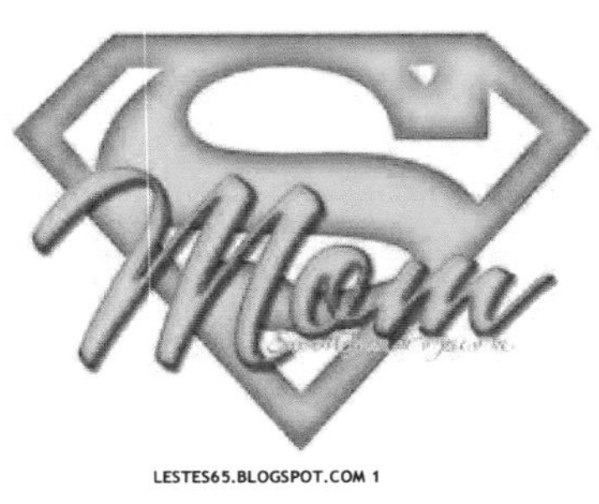

LESTES65.BLOGSPOT.COM 1

You know your child better than anyone. You know the child's habits, schedule, things the child likes and dislikes. You know that your child has a diagnosis and cannot take care of him/herself. You are the person that will speak on your child's behalf when it comes to addressing issues at school or with medical care. The best thing is that when you're dealing with issues regarding your child , your participation comes from the heart, its genuine. This is what makes you your child's best advocate. Advocates are needed for various issues, however, we are going to focus on advocating for children diagnosed with Sickle Cell. You're probably like "aduh!" Well I just want to be clear. The tools you are going to need to be an effective advocate include:

1. Learn how to communicate effectively. What does this mean? This simply means that it would be best if you expressed yourself clearly. This also means that you will hear things that you don't agree with but it is ok, just be attentive and listen. If what you hear angers you, remove yourself from the situation and/or conversation and give yourself time to think about what angered you and how to effectively deal with the issue head on. Don't be afraid to ask others for advice. Two heads are always better than one.
2. What is the issue that you are advocating for? Having a child with a chronic illness pretty much guarantees that you will find a few things to advocate for. Know what you want first.
3. Do your homework! Research, read and learn everything you can about your child's illness.

SPRINGTOWNISD.NET 1

4. Familiarize yourself with the Rules & Regulations, Standard Operating Procedures and laws that pertain to your issue. Dont forget to look for potential loopholes. It's not hard to do, trust me!
5. Form positive relationships with any professional that will be working with your child. There will be some that you absolutely can't stand, it's ok, just pretend. Your child can only benefit. Remember you will get more with sugar than vinegar.
6. Document! Document! Document! As I mentioned, record every aspect of your child's medical care. Request and obtain copies of reports. Be sure to have your paperwork in order (dates will probably be the easiest).

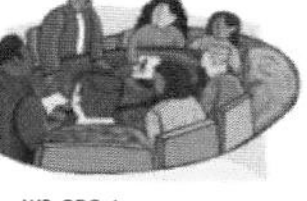
W3.ORG 1

7. Attend all meetings pertaining to your child. There will be times that you

are physically unable to attend, when that happens, request that they conference the meeting. Simply put, they will have a speaker phone and call you up. Everyone else involved will be able to speak. Also with today's technology it may be possible to attend via webcam.

8. Don't be afraid to ask questions. There will be times when "something" just doesn't sit right with you. When this happens do not be afraid to ask questions and don't be intimidated or embarrassed. You will have some professionals that will talk past you, above you or at you but not to you. When this happens bring them down a notch and let them know in a cordial tone that you need clarification. This is your child. Do not walk away pretending you know what just went on if you really don't. The only dumb question is the one that goes unasked!
9. Don't be afraid to say "no." If you don't agree with something you are not obligated to just go with the flow of things. Explain why your uncomfortable with whatever it is and request that the issue be examined.
10. Use technology to keep everyone on the same page. Be sure to have the email addresses of every professional involved in your child's care. In today's world it is easier to reach people using email. Almost every professional has a blackberry or iPhone. When you send an email it goes to their phone immediately and they are more likely to read the email instantly. I know that a call reaches them immediately but they will not always answer their phone. PS. Always blind copy yourself on every email!
11. You are your child's hero. Currently I keep my child out of certain issues that I believe will upset her or issues that I feel are not age appropriate. I am going to let my child be a child because she only lives once. As she ages, I will involve her more and allow her to express how she feels about certain things. My goal is to teach her how to advocate for herself, I will not be around forever. This is just my approach. We all know that every parent raises their child different. This is a parental choice.

PIXMAC.COM 1

Dear Mom, Please Don't Forget to take Care of Yourself!

What you need to know

- ✓ It's easy to slip into depression
- ✓ You must take care of yourself

What you need to do

- ✓ *Join support groups*

  Joining a support group will prove to be beneficial in the long run. There are many support groups online and offline. You will meet people that truly understand what you're going through because they have walked miles in your shoes. We all need someone to lean on.

Take time off-take a vacation

No matter the vacation, big or small, you need to take one! It is unhealthy to go on and on and on without a break. Having a child diagnosed with a chronic illness can be stressful and become more stressful by the day. Trust me, a vacation will do you some good! After all, how effective can you be if you are a total wreck? Holding fears, anger or sadness in can kill you.

Taking care of yourself is needed to Take Care of your Child!!!!!

I was so guilty of this. Who would of thought that I would forget to attend to my needs. Taking care of myself never occurred to me. I was so wrapped up in my child's care that it became obsessive. Can you blame me? I was one of those mothers who wanted instant results at any cost, even if it meant sacrificing my personal well-being . I am involved in every aspect of her medical care, schooling, recreation and everything else.

What I began to notice was that I was exhausted and when like this could I really provide the quality care my child needed? Taking care of myself meant joining support groups and being able to talk about my anxieties and reservations. I met some really good people and we have formed lasting relationships. Most importantly I realized that my child was very perceptive. She was able to sense when something was wrong or when I was sad. The last thing that I needed was to have her worried about me.

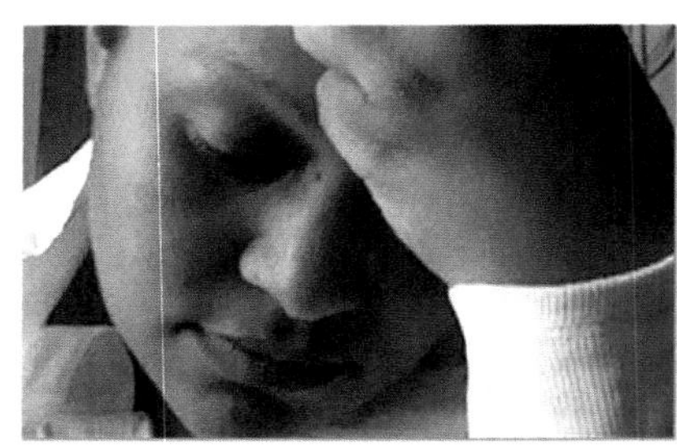

You may be the strongest person in the world and considered to be the "rock" of the family. You are probably the person that everyone calls when something goes wrong. It can become overwhelming because the "rock" has issues to. Who is going to be the shoulder to lean on when the "rock" is not feeling so awesome?

Taking care of a child diagnosed with Sickle Cell is a lot of work. If you don't have a support network in place it becomes overwhelming, and quickly I might add. It is a life long disease that can create pain and chaos in your child's life at anytime. As caregivers we must be "at the ready" at all times, 24 hours a day, 365 days a year. We fulfill several different roles and must assume our position when that particular role is needed.

Is Your Legal House in Order?

This is a very touchy topic but there is no other way to say it, Plan! Plan! Plan! Anything can happen to you at anytime. If you are the primary caretaker of the child then be sure to have all of your legal documents in place. It is like having a plan B. If something happens to you, plan B should instantly be in full effect. Just ask yourself …

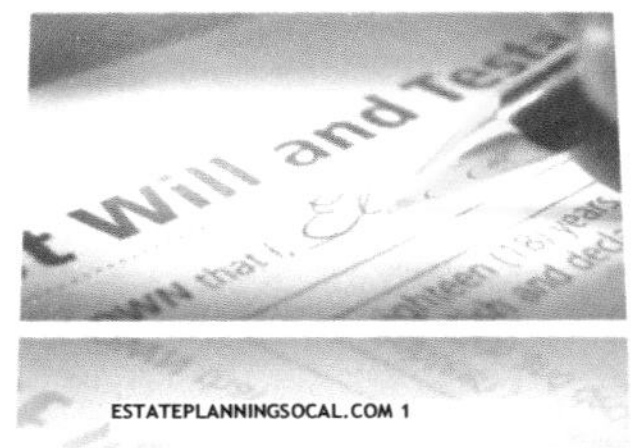

1. Who is going to take my child? Can I depend on the other parent?
2. My child is underage, so how will my child live in my house?
3. Do I have an Advanced Medical Directive in place?
4. Do I have a Durable Power of Attorney for Healthcare in place?

If you found that you didn't have the answer to one of these questions please get your legal documents in order and plan for your child's future care. If you don't know where to start you have a few options. You can do it the old fashioned way and go to your phonebook. You may want to look up your local "Legal Aide." You can also go to the yellow pages and search for "legal," and you will find many attorneys there that offer free consultations, will point you in the right direction and some attorneys may be willing to help you "pro bono."(Free of charge). Some documents that you may find useful are:

1. Revocable Trust
2. Will/Pour Over Will
3. Durable Power of Attorney for Healthcare
4. Advanced Directive Instructions
5. Financial Power of Attorney
6. Life Insurance Policy -be sure all beneficiaries are up to date
7. Mortgage Insurance

Chapter 7

Maintaining a Healthy Family

The Parent Trap

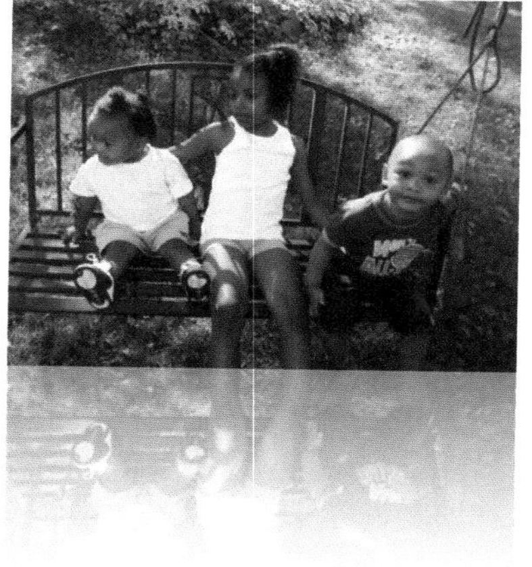

Caring for your child requires vigilance and tenacity. The situation can become obsessive rather quickly—especially in the beginning—and you can easily lose your way in caring for your other children. As a result, your other children can suddenly find themselves receiving a lot less attention from you. An integral part of providing care for your child is to safeguard the overall health of your entire family. It is important that you find and maintain a balance between caring for all of your children. In your quest to preserve this balance there will be times when you will feel as though you are walking a tightrope while juggling sticks of dynamite—with the fusses lit! But trust me, it will become easier as time progresses.

Go Fish

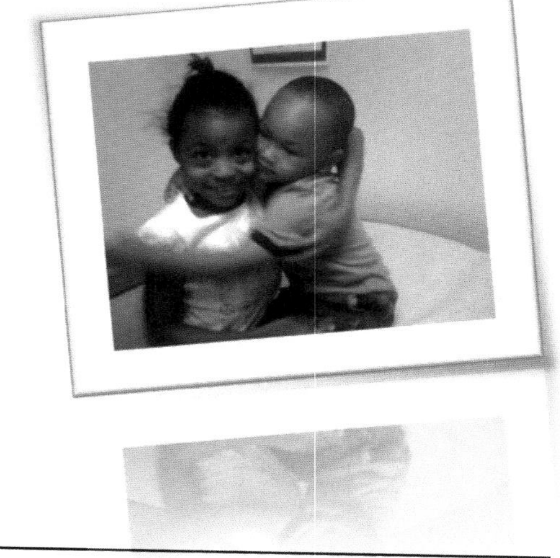

Haven't we all played this children's card game? As parents we sometimes forget what it means to be a kid and yet, key to maintaining a healthy family is remembering how to do just that. A happy family is a healthy family! The easiest way to give equal attention to your children is by devising activities which involve the entire family. Here are some tips for family fun time:

- ✓ Movie Night
- ✓ Baking Cookies

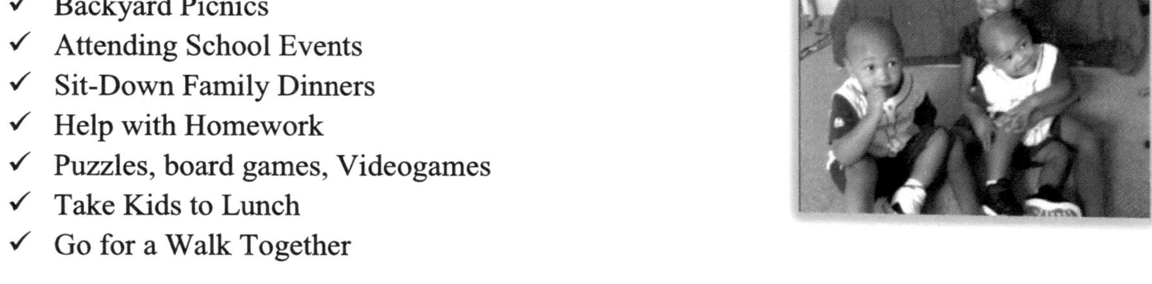

- ✓ Backyard Picnics
- ✓ Attending School Events
- ✓ Sit-Down Family Dinners
- ✓ Help with Homework
- ✓ Puzzles, board games, Videogames
- ✓ Take Kids to Lunch
- ✓ Go for a Walk Together

Of course, all of your children are going to need some alone time and you might want to consider going for walks or doing some activity that is meaningful to that particular child. You also want to be sure to talk to your children, find out what's going on at school with their friends. Stay involved in their lives. Also, be sure to explain to your children (if they are of age) the nature of their brother/sisters illness and why you must focus extra attention on them. In no way does it mean you love them (the others) any less.

References

A.D.A.M., Inc., Initials. (2010, November 15). *Bile*. Retrieved from http://www.nlm.nih.gov/medlineplus/ency/article/002237.htm

A.D.A.M., Inc., Initials. (2004). *Sickle-cell disease*. Retrieved from http://adam.about.com/reports/000058_5.htm

Autism Society, Initials. (n.d.). *Individualized education plan (iep)*. Retrieved from http://www.autism-society.org/site/PageServer?pagename=life_edu_IEP

Cedars-Sinai Medical Center, Initials. (2010). *Doctor online referral schedule a callback transcranial doppler*. Retrieved from http://www.cedars-sinai.edu/Patients/Programs-and-Services/Neurology/Diagnostic-Services/Transcranial-Doppler.aspx

Crowley, C.F. (2010, July 24). *Barriers leave blacks vulnerable to cancer*. Retrieved from http://albarchive.merlinone.net/mweb/wmsql.wm.request?oneimage&imageid=11464181

Education Center, Initials. (n.d.). *504 plan v. iep*. Retrieved from http://www.ed-center.com/504

Family Practice Notebook, LLC, Initials. (2010). *Priapism in sickle cell anemia*. Retrieved from http://www.fpnotebook.com/hemeonc/Hemoglobin/PrpsmInSckIClAnm.htm

Gardner MD, FACP, FACG , P.W., & Waldstreicher MD, FACG , S. (1993). *Gallstones*. Retrieved from http://www.gastro.com/gastro/gallstones.aspx

March of Dimes, Initials. (2004, August). *Sickle cell disease*. Retrieved from http://health.msn.com/kids-health/articlepage.aspx?cp-documentid=100169868

Medical College of Georgia, Initials. (2010). *Comprehenisve sickle cell center*. Retrieved from http://www.mcg.edu/centers/sicklecell/

Morris, Ph.D, J.D. (n.d.). *Does the gallbladder have a necessary function?*. Retrieved from http://www.icr.org/index.php?module=articles&action=view&ID=17

My Optum Health , Initials. (n.d.). *Sickle cell disease*. Retrieved from http://www.myoptumhealth.com/portal/DiseasesandConditions/item/Sickle+cell+disease

National Institute of Health. NIH Publication No. 96-4057. November 1996.

New York State Department of Health, Professional Medical Conduct and Physician Discipline. (2008). *How to choose the right physician - how to tell us if you don't* New York State: Retrieved from http://www.health.state.ny.us/publications/1444/

Privacy Rights Clearinghouse / UCAN , Initials. (2010, September). *Fact sheet 8a: hipaa basics: medical privacy in the electronic age* . Retrieved from http://www.privacyrights.org/fs/fs8a-hipaa.htm

U.S. Department of Health and Human Services, Indian Helath Service. (2008). *helath insurance portability and accountability act* Retrieved from http://www.hipaa.ihs.gov/index.cfm?module=faq

CPSIA information can be obtained
at www.ICGtesting.com
Printed in the USA
LVIW021448251012
304451LV00006B

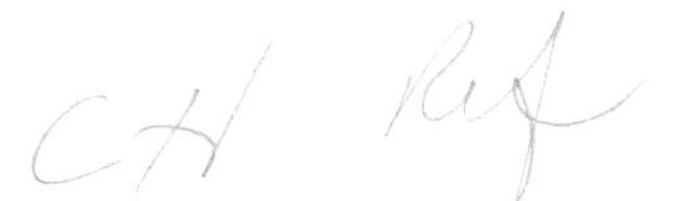

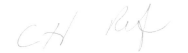